Weight Loss Cure: Melt Fat Naturally (2025)

Your Guide to Cellular Health: Unlocking the Science of Longevity and Joy (2024)

The Truth About COVID-19: Exposing The Great Reset, Lockdowns, Vaccine Passports, and the New Normal (2021, with Ronnie Cummins)

EMF*D: 5G, Wi-Fi & Cell Phones: Hidden Harms and How to Protect Yourself (2020)

KetoFast: Rejuvenate Your Health with a Step-by-Step Guide to Timing Your Ketogenic Meals (2019)

Fat for Fuel: A Revolutionary Diet to Combat Cancer, Boost Brain Power, and Increase Your Energy (2017)

Effortless Healing: 9 Simple Ways to Sidestep Illness, Shed Excess Weight, and Help Your Body Fix Itself (2015)

Dark Deception: Discover the Truths About the Benefits of Sunlight Exposure (2008)

Generation XL: Raising Healthy, Intelligent Kids in a High-Tech, Junk-Food World (2007)

Take Control of Your Health (2007, with Dr. Kendra Degen Pearsall)

The Great Bird Flu Hoax: The Truth They Don't Want You To Know About The "Next Big Pandemic" (2006, with Pam Killeen)

Sweet Deception: Why Splenda, NutraSweet, and the FDA May Be Hazardous to Your Health (2006, with Dr. Kendra Degen Pearsall)

The No-Grain Diet: Conquer Carbohydrate Addiction and Stay Slim for Life (2003, with Dr. Alison Rose Levy)

GUT CURE

STOP THE ROT

Restore Your Body
From the **Inside Out**

GUT CURE

STOP THE ROT

Restore Your Body
From the Inside Out

Dr. Mercola

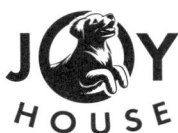

JOY
HOUSE

Hardcover ISBN: 978-1-965429-08-2

eBook ISBN: 978-1-965429-09-9

PUBLISHED BY
Joy House Publishing
125 SW 3rd Place, Suite 200, Cape Coral, FL 33991

Joyhousepublishing.com
For rights and permissions please contact media@mercola.com

Book and cover design by Alexia Garaventa

Manufactured in the United States of America

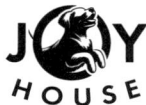

CONTENTS

Note to Readers

The author of this book does not advocate the use of any particular form of health care for all individuals but believes that the facts, figures, and knowledge presented herein should be available to every person concerned with improving his or her state of health. This book is not intended to replace the advice and treatment of the reader's personal physician or health-care provider. Any use of the information set forth herein is entirely at the reader's discretion.

The author and publisher are not responsible for any adverse effects or consequences resulting from the use of any of the preparations or procedures described in this book. This book is based upon the author's own opinion and theories. The reader should always consult with his or her own health-care practitioner before taking any medicine or dietary, nutritional, herbal, or homeopathic supplement, or beginning or stopping any therapy. The author is not intending to provide a substitute for the reader's personal medical advice and makes no warranty whatsoever, expressed or implied, with respect to any product, device, or therapy. No statement in this book has been reviewed or approved by the United States Food and Drug Administration or the Federal Trade Commission. Readers should use their own judgment in consultation with a holistic medical expert or their personal physician or health-care provider for specific applications to their health-care needs.

Preface

I never set out to become a "gut detective," but in hindsight, the path was always leading there. Even in medical school, I was known as "Dr. Fiber" for my passion for food as medicine and whole-body healing. From the start of my career as a doctor of osteopathic medicine (DO), my mission was to uncover the true root causes of illness—not to medicate symptoms into silence. Early on, I saw that drugs didn't resolve the chronic issues my patients faced. I wanted to free them from dependence on prescriptions that offered little real progress. What I didn't fully grasp back then was just how central the gut was to nearly every chronic disease I was trying to treat. Over the years, it became impossible to ignore: Gut health wasn't just part of the picture; it was often the starting point.

What began as a search for answers in complex chronic conditions soon revealed something even more pervasive. The gut wasn't just at the root of diagnosable diseases but also the missing link in the everyday symptoms that so many people silently endure: fatigue without cause; brain fog with no explanation; a vague sense that something just isn't right.

Today we face a quiet epidemic: patients who look healthy on paper—normal labs, normal weight, diligent with their exercise—yet they still feel exhausted, achy, foggy, and oddly older than their years.

No textbook can explain why a marathon runner can barely climb the stairs at night or why a health-conscious mother feels spent after an ordinary breakfast. But when you dig deeper, a pattern emerges: Their guts are inflamed, starved, and pleading for help.

That realization sent me deep into the science—into the microbiome, short-chain fatty acids (or what I refer to as Gut Gems in my *Cure* book series), and the hidden damage caused by modern seed oils and industrial additives. One thread led to another, and the pattern became clear: The gut isn't just a digestive organ; it's the body's command center for energy, immunity, metabolism, and mood. And today it's under siege. The trillions of microbes we rely on to keep us well—once nourished by real food and unpolluted air—are now suffocating under a relentless assault of linoleic acid, emulsifiers, pesticides, and plastic residues.

I wrote *Gut Cure* and divided it into two accessible volumes because most people have never heard that story. They are told their fatigue is the result of "just getting older," their brain fog is caused by "too much screen time," their restless sleep is "busy modern life." They are offered pills, patches, and injections that muffle symptoms while the underlying fire keeps smoldering. I refuse to accept that future for my clients, my family, or you.

You will not find rigid meal plans, calorie math, or shaming language on these pages. What you will find is a map: the science of how butyrate and its companion Gut Gems repair the intestinal lining; the truth about polyunsaturated seed oils that headline as "heart-healthy" while crippling microbial diversity; the elegant loops between your colon and brain that decide whether you reach for a pastry at 3:00 p.m. or breeze past it without a second thought.

You will also meet Mara, a fictional yet all-too-real composite of countless patients I have treated over the course of my clinical career. Her wins and missteps are here to keep the research grounded in lived experience—because data alone rarely sparks lasting change. Stories do. If you recognize yourself in Mara's struggles, then you're one step closer to understanding what's really behind your symptoms—and to finally knowing where to begin.

Most of all, I wrote this book to hand the levers of control back to you. The food industry spends billions teaching you to doubt your cravings for genuine nourishment and to silence your body's protest with "better-for-you" snacks that are anything but. The *Gut Cure* volumes are my answer to that noise—a practical, hopeful guide to lowering the toxic load, reviving microbial allies, and letting your gut resume its role as the quiet powerhouse it was designed to be.

Change doesn't start with perfection—it starts with one small step. Maybe it's swapping canola oil for butter. Maybe it's pausing to read an ingredient label. Maybe it's simply paying attention when your gut whispers, instead of waiting for it to scream. However small it seems, that first step matters. Because when you show up for your gut, your microbes will show up for you.

Whether you are a clinician searching for root-cause answers, a weekend athlete sidelined by unexplained aches, or a parent who simply wants energy that lasts past bedtime stories, this book is for you. I have condensed decades of clinical observation, hundreds of peer-reviewed studies, and my own hard-earned lessons into these chapters. My hope is that by the final page, you'll no longer feel like a passive passenger in your health journey but the one confidently charting the course—map and compass in hand, feet on solid ground. *Gut Cure* isn't just a title—it's your invitation to understand what's really going on beneath the surface. Let's dig in.

Introduction: Your Microbiome Deserves the Spotlight

Meet Mara. As a lively gym-goer and nutrition enthusiast, Mara puts her health first. She's only in her forties now, but regardless of her commitment to exercise and health, she has suffered from body aches and inconsistent energy for almost a decade now. And lately her symptoms have gotten even worse.

At the gym, Mara deadlifts her own body weight and earns nods from fellow lifters who admire her grit. Her kitchen is a testament to "clean eating," by fitness magazine standards; it features lean chicken, protein shakes, granola bars, salad ingredients, low-fat dressings, and her trusted "heart-healthy" canola oil. Mara is proud of her discipline and certain she has positively transformed her lifestyle, especially her diet. Since her body aches have grown worse, so have her mood swings, energy crashes, and gut troubles. Mara blames it on aging and possibly overtraining. She would never believe her diet had anything to do with it. Chasing diet fads and trends, however, has hidden the real trouble brewing in Mara's gut.

Mara's story is our gateway into this book. At the end of each chapter, you will meet her as someone whose struggles might echo your own. Although she is a fictional character, Mara faces real-life patterns that I've seen over and over in counseling patients and simply observing human behavior. Her journey brings the science of the gut to everyday life, showing us what happens when gut dysfunction is misunderstood, ignored, or misdiagnosed. Most importantly, Mara shows us what it looks like to turn things around.

I'm a physician, but this isn't another dry, clinical guide. I've blended science with storytelling because facts alone rarely motivate significant changes. We need to turn ideas into actions, and we are more likely to act when we are emotionally engaged with what we are learning. If Mara's story clicks with you and helps you see your own path more clearly, then perhaps real changes will follow and make all the difference in your life.

Mara's gut, like yours, is a teeming city of trillions of microbes. If she has given any thought to her gut's microscopic residents, she's assumed they just handle digestion, but they're far more impactful than that. They adjust her immune defenses, affect her mood, and aid her stamina.

Every bite Mara takes casts a vote on which microbes thrive and which falter in her gut. Like so many others, Mara thinks she's eating the healthiest foods, but most of her meals are built around the wrong fats. The low-fat dressings Mara uses tout "heart-healthy" sunflower, safflower, corn, and soybean oils. But she's about to learn that those unstable oils are packed with linoleic acid (LA), an omega-6 polyunsaturated fat. I call these fats PUFS throughout this book—a term that refers specifically to the excess omega-6 seed oils driving today's health crisis, not to all polyunsaturated fats, which also include the more beneficial omega-3s.

No matter how many times you may see or hear them described in positive terms such as "heart healthy," PUFS in excess are toxic to the gut. Why? They help the wrong microbes. In simple terms, PUFS allow harmful bacteria to flourish so much that they overpower the beneficial microbes your gut needs to keep your body in check.

That said, in tiny doses, PUFS are essential to your body. Unfortunately, modern processed foods are jam-packed with these fats. Crisp munchies, cooking oils, and countless packaged goods contain PUFS—much more than Mara's gut, or yours—can handle.

Ironically, she is far more careful about her diet than almost everyone she knows. For one thing, Mara limits how much sugar she consumes. Also, as someone who works out to build and maintain muscle tone, she eats plenty of lean protein. PUFS, however, are stealthy. They sneak in through many packaged foods and cause gut inflammation.

In time, Mara will learn that while PUFS may hide in all kinds of foods, her body will always expose them. Bloating and energy crashes are her main clues! Upon realizing that whatever she has eaten contains excessive PUFS, Mara will begin to track down their sources and swap them for much healthier, more satisfying alternatives.

Until then, Mara must face the ramifications of other dietary aspects, like skimping on fiber. Her salads may look healthy, but ingredients such as lettuce and celery are mostly water, which don't provide much fuel for her gut microbes. Without enough fermentable fiber, her good gut bacteria are starving and unable to churn out short-chain fatty acids (SCFAs), or what we'll call *Gut Gems* in this book.

Gut Gems are tiny powerhouses that are made when microbes feast on fiber from beans, colorful vegetables, and whole grains. They ensure everything runs smoothly. They keep inflammation at bay, fine-tune immunity, and help Mara rebound from stress. When they are in short supply, chaos ensues in the gut.

Through Mara's journey, we will trace how PUFS and other modern traps—such as a lack of fiber, exposure to industrial toxins, and misguided diet trends—derail her balance. We will also uncover how small, deliberate shifts can bring her gut—and yours—back to life.

Most importantly, as you'll learn in chapter 1, your gut and its inhabitants are unique to you. Mara's discoveries may guide you, but you may need to adjust her approach or seek additional solutions from a trusted medical professional. This book is your invitation to understand your gut's unique ecosystem and to nurture it. With Mara—who is flawed, determined, and utterly relatable—leading the charge, we will explore why your microbial world matters and learn how to shield it from the everyday assaults of modern living.

The Path to Gut Health

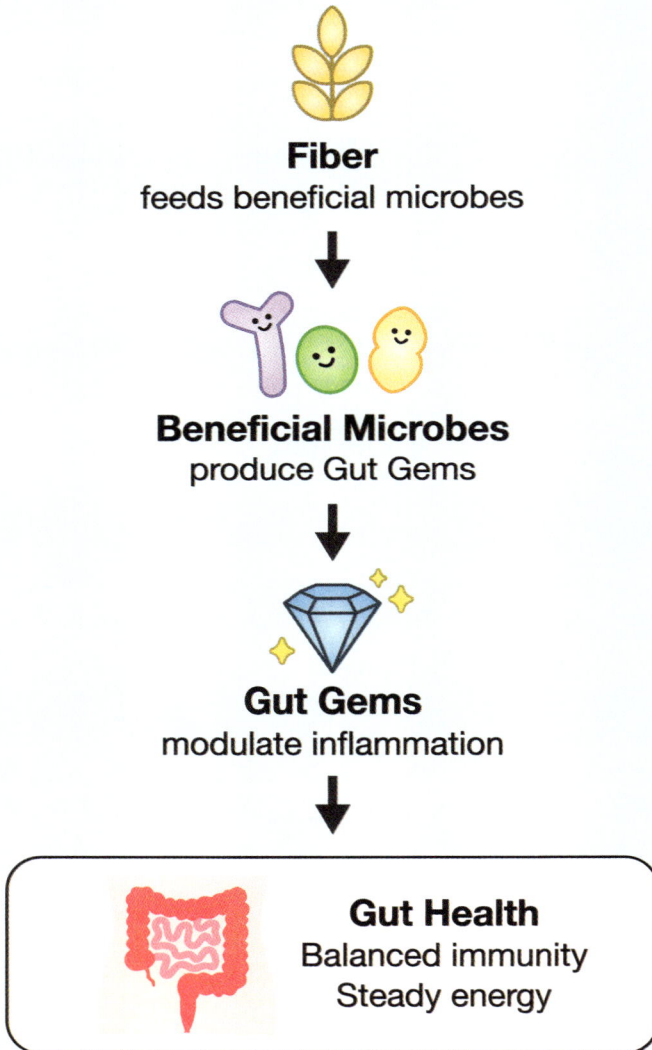

Fiber
feeds beneficial microbes

Beneficial Microbes
produce Gut Gems

Gut Gems
modulate inflammation

Gut Health
Balanced immunity
Steady energy

Fig. 1: When beneficial microbes feast on fiber, they produce short-chain fatty acids (SCFAs)—referred to as Gut Gems in this book—which control inflammation and promote a healthy gut that boosts immunity and energy.

CHAPTER 1

Introduction to Your Gut Microbiome

Your gut microbiome is a unique ecosystem. Imagine a vast microbial city with trillions of inhabitants. It is shaped by diet, lifestyle, and genetics, much like a personal health signature. When balanced, this complex, interdependent community of bacteria supports digestion, immunity, and well-being by producing vital compounds and regulating inflammation. With our modern diet, however, the microbiome can easily get out of balance.

Microbial Diversity Is Key

The gut has many different species of bacteria, each with unique strengths and capabilities. A diverse mix of bacterial types makes your digestion smooth, so your immune system functions optimally.

The human microbiome is made up of three main phyla, or groups of gut microbes, and they serve diverse structural, protective, and metabolic functions:

- **Bacteroidetes** play a role in breaking down complex carbohydrates and producing vitamins, as well as helping to regulate the immune system.
- **Firmicutes** are centrally involved in glucose, insulin, and metabolism, and are useful in helping your gut break down sugars and carbohydrates from the foods you eat.

> • **Actinobacteria** digest complex carbohydrates, produce vitamins B12 and K2, and protect against pathogens.

As unique to you as your fingerprints, your microbial makeup has been shaped from the moment you were born. Infants are exposed to their mother's bacterial population through childbirth and breastfeeding. The mother's bacteria colonize the child's gastrointestinal tract and continue to influence their bacterial makeup well into adulthood. If you were born through cesarean surgery and/or were fed formula as a baby, your microbiome may not be as diverse as someone who was born vaginally and/or breastfed.

Antibiotics also influence your bacterial population. While these medications help kill harmful bacteria, they also eradicate beneficial ones. All told, a course of antibiotics can cut microbial richness by 30 percent. In fact, the reason for adding probiotic- or prebiotic-rich foods to your diet if you are prescribed antibiotics is to help reseed your gut with healthy microbes. Fermented foods such as yogurt, kefir, kimchi, and sauerkraut also contain microorganisms and compounds that support microbial diversity.

If you've ever blamed your tummy troubles on bad luck, think again. The balance of your gut microbes can influence everything from gas, bloating, constipation, and diarrhea to those daily energy crashes and annoying sniffles that crop up. Sure, it could be the office air conditioner or allergy season, but chances are your microbes have more influence over how you feel than you realize.

A balanced gut is your body's VIP security team on standby; it defuses problems before they escalate. An imbalanced gut, in contrast, struggles to keep small triggers in check. Before you know it, they turn into full-blown issues like skin flare-ups, mood swings, and body aches.

Small shifts in your diet can have a big impact on your mood and energy in positive and negative ways. Ever notice how a single weekend of better eating can make you feel like you can conquer the world? That's your gut microbes responding to the good nutrition you finally supplied. Just as quickly, however, a "cheat week" can make you wonder why your energy is in the gutter. Again, it's your gut responding, only not so politely, to the loads of junk food you just ate. Shifts in how you feel throughout your body happen because gut microbes send out chemical messages that influence your immune cells, adjust your stress responses, and shape how you absorb nutrients. The communication is so seamless that you would have no reason to think of it—until something goes haywire.

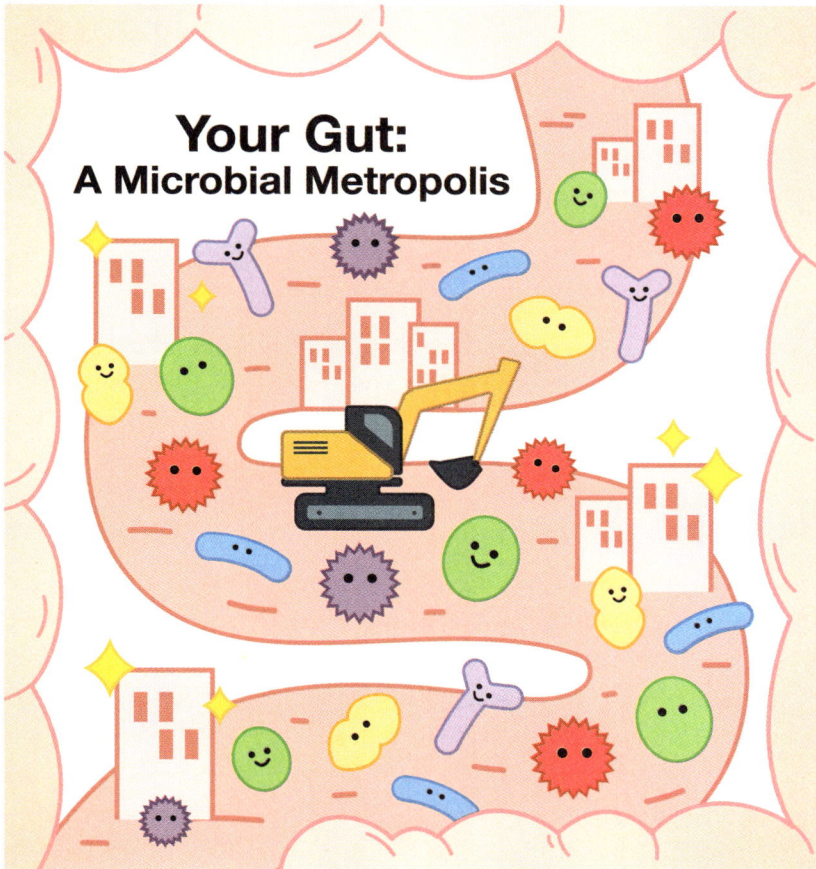

Your Gut:
A Microbial Metropolis

Fig. 2: When everything is working well, your gut is home to a thriving population of diverse microbes, each with their own important roles to play.

The Fiber Paradox

Your friendly gut microbes love to munch on fiber. When they have plenty of fiber to feast on, they produce amazing substances called short-chain fatty acids (SCFAs), or what we are referring to as Gut Gems. Soluble fiber dissolves in water and directly feeds your gut microbes, while insoluble fiber adds bulk and keeps things moving. Insoluble fiber can also support gut microbes, though typically to a lesser extent. While there are many different SCFAs, one of the most important, which you'll learn more about in chapters 2 and 3, is butyrate (BYOO-tih-rate). Butyrate is a star among Gut Gems because it helps the lining of your colon stay strong. As a result, it reduces inflammation, regulates bowel movements, and helps prevent colon cancer and inflammatory bowel disease (IBD).

But loading up on fiber won't produce Gut Gems if your gut is in poor shape. While fiber is great for your gut, it requires the right balance of gut bacteria to be beneficial. If your gut has too many harmful microbes and not enough beneficial ones, fiber ends up feeding the bad bacteria and fostering their growth instead. This situation is known as the fiber paradox. In that case, piling on fiber can cause uncomfortable bloating or unpredictable digestion, leaving you baffled as to why the "miracle cure" of fiber isn't living up to the hype.

The solution is to shore up your gut environment first. That could mean stepping back from daily onslaughts of industrial toxins, especially PUFS, that can tip your microbial balance in the wrong direction. It may also mean looking at postbiotic and probiotic *Akkermansia* supplements. The purpose of such supplements is to help you repair your gut and reseed it with Gut Gem-producing bacteria. Once the balance of your gut microbiome is restored, fiber will fuel the beneficial microbes that produce Gut Gems in greater volumes that help you feel centered and strong.

The Fiber Paradox: Why More Isn't Always Better (Initially)

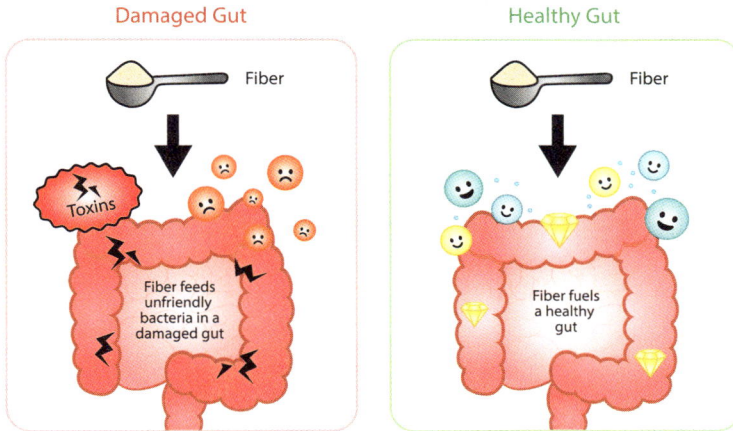

Fig. 3: If your gut is already struggling, adding more fiber may cause more upset. As you reduce your consumption of toxins, such as PUFS, your gut can tolerate more fiber and produce more Gut Gems.

In Case You Skipped the Intro, We're Talking About PUFS—Again

Throughout this book, I will mention a certain type of fat called linoleic acid, which is an omega-6 polyunsaturated fatty acid. The term *acid* here is easy to misunderstand. In real foods, these acids are usually bound in triglycerides, a type of fat. Therefore they do not behave the way acids would in a lab test tube. So, for easier understanding, I'm calling them PUFS, short for polyunsaturated fats, which includes linoleic acid.

You will find PUFS in everything from everyday cooking oils (such as corn, safflower, sunflower, and canola oils) to processed foods and restaurant meals. If the acronym *PUFS* triggers images of crispy cheese puffs, that's right on the money. Tons of munchable snacks rely on these oils.

A small amount of PUFS is okay, but go past that "tiny amount" threshold and your microbiome can shift in the wrong direction. Don't be surprised if this happens when you believe you are doing everything right and eating healthy foods.

Let's look at the chemistry behind why PUFS cause problems. Such fats are called *poly*unsaturated because they have multiple double bonds in their molecular structure. Those double bonds, however, are fragile and break apart easily when exposed to heat, light, or oxygen. When that happens, the fats oxidize and turn into reactive compounds that damage your cells, irritate your gut lining, and disrupt microbial balance.

In contrast, saturated fats have no double bonds. As a result, their structure is more stable and less likely to break down under stress. That's why fats such as coconut oil, butter, and beef tallow hold up better, both during cooking and inside your body. They don't turn rancid as quickly, and they don't trigger the same level of oxidative stress as PUFS do. In short, PUFS create metabolic chaos. Saturated fats offer stability that your body can count on.

PUFS also disrupt the microbial balance in your gut through a system of competition. Picture your gut as a tranquil pond. Fish, plants, and algae all live together in a stable ecosystem. Now imagine someone pours in a chemical that makes one type of algae explode in number. In turn, the fish and plants die out. In a similar way, PUFS can skew your microbial diversity. Beneficial microbes that produce Gut Gems may get crowded out by opportunistic strains that thrive in the new environment. The results can manifest in the symptoms we've mentioned, such as feeling bloated after meals, noticing your moods are more erratic, or developing a rash.

Small Steps to Swap PUFS for Stable Fat

Let's shift gears to help you eat in a way that doesn't revolve around fiber. Especially take note if your gut is currently in no shape to handle it. Instead of debating health trends that would tell you to increase your fiber, we will focus on one simple action: swapping out PUFS-filled foods for saturated fat–based alternatives. My suggestion is to choose butter, ghee, tallow, and coconut oil. No matter which one(s) you pick, the idea is to reduce the daily barrage of harmful fats. As a result, you will give your gut a breather so it can create an environment that is more conducive to Gut Gem production.

First, without overthinking everything you eat, mentally review your typical meals and snacks. Starting with snacks, do you have a go-to brand of chips? If you checked the ingredients, would they contain PUFS? Are you buying a store-bought dressing? Is soybean oil a main ingredient? If you desire a crunchy granola bar, how will its ingredients treat your gut? Now pick one or two items that you can easily replace.

For example, if you find that your potato chips were fried in seed oils, try a root vegetable mix cooked in coconut oil. Instead of store-bought salad dressing, whisk up your own recipe. For a zesty, healthy option, use liquefied coconut oil, balsamic vinegar, a splash of lemon juice, raw honey, and your choice of herbs. Replace PUFS-filled granola bars with homemade versions, perhaps using coconut flakes, cacao nibs, and a touch of honey.

Next, pay attention to how your body responds over the course of a week with fewer PUFS in your meals. Maybe your afternoon energy is steady. Maybe your digestion feels calmer.

If snacks made with stable, saturated fats feel easier on your system, keep going. Try sautéing your vegetables in coconut oil, scrambling eggs in beef tallow, or greasing baking pans with butter instead of canola oil spray. Before long, small adjustments like this will become second nature, and your gut will reward you for your efforts.

Every small win contributes to a gut environment that's more receptive to other improvements that you may introduce down the line. You can also explore adding C15:0 (the essential odd-chain saturated fat highlighted in *Fat Cure* and covered here in chapter 19) to further support a gut environment that keeps your beneficial microbes thriving.

Mapping Your Microbes: A Visual Guide to Their Interactions

Imagine your gut as a giant intersection of roads with each microbe type as a little car. Depending on the fuel you feed them, the cars can merge, turn, or leave the highway entirely.

Now picture a big sign that reads "Gut Gem Production This Way." Each fiber-based meal leads your beneficial microbes down the Gut Gem route. As a result, these microbes churn out a stable supply of protective, inflammation-cooling SCFAs (Gut Gems). If you are consistent with consuming the right amount of fiber and keeping your PUFS intake low, you will have a flowing intersection with minimal traffic jams. However, if your daily meals revolve around processed snacks or questionable cooking oils, your microbes might take a wrong turn and end up stuck in a congested zone of harmful bacterial strains. As they multiply, metabolic gridlock worsens.

It might sound silly to think of your gut as a mini city, bustling with traffic, but the mental image can help you visualize why variety and moderation matter. Too much of one thing—be it refined fructose (a favorite food of unfriendly bacteria), PUFS, or antibiotics—can create a pileup that takes time to clear. Meanwhile, a stable intake of fiber (once your gut health is in a good place), saturated fats, and conscious meal planning open multiple lanes for Gut Gem production, keeping everything from your digestion to your mood running smoothly.

Gut Microbe Traffic Flow

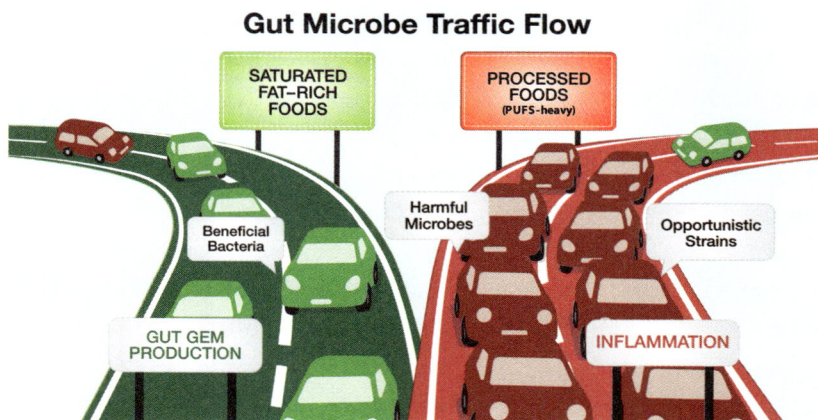

Fig. 4: Because PUFS encourage the growth of unfriendly bacteria, switching to saturated fats is a great way to nourish gut health.

On any day, if you catch yourself about to grab something heavily processed, consider asking, "Will the ingredients direct traffic the right way or clog things up?" The point is to remember that each choice has a consequence for your microbial traffic pattern. Over time, your awareness alone can steer you toward more beneficial decisions, even when convenience foods tempt you.

If you slip up, remember that your gut is adaptable. A weekend party's temptation or some junk food while traveling may cause a temporary uptick in less-friendly microbes. But as soon as you get back to your routine by avoiding PUFS and refined fructose, the traffic flow can recalibrate.

Take an Easy Gut-Health Quiz to See How You're Doing

If all this talk about microbes and Gut Gems feels a bit abstract, you may wonder, "Where do I even start?" That is where the Gut-Health Quiz comes in. Consider it a friendly self-check that you can do without any medical equipment.

For the next week, keep a mini food journal. Simply list what you ate for your key meals and snacks. Also record whether you used saturated fats such as butter or ghee or ended up with PUFS-based products.

Also note how your digestion and mood felt after each meal. Did you experience bloating, sharp energy dips, or odd cravings? Did you feel surprisingly full and satisfied? Were you hungry again in an hour? Your personal investigation can reveal important patterns. For example, perhaps you always felt sluggish on the days you had store-bought salad dressing. If the bottle was loaded with PUFS, you will know why!

Next, ask yourself if you have recently taken antibiotics or if you skipped fiber-laden foods more often than not. You can go one step further and incorporate observations about stress levels or your daily water intake. Maybe you'll notice you felt drained on the days you didn't hydrate or lethargic when you stressed over a work deadline. Taking notes allows you to see how everything—diet, stress, hydration—intertwines.

Putting the puzzle pieces together can highlight areas that are working well and those that might need an overhaul. Once you know your baseline, it's also easier to set realistic goals.

The quiz does not have a pass or fail mark. Think of it as an opportunity to get an eye-opening look at how your diet treats your microbiome. From there, you can consider which adjustments you would like to try and potentially make a real difference in how you feel.

My Gut-Health Quiz Log

Date	Meal/Snack	Key Ingredients	Digestion Notes	Mood/Energy Notes	Other Factors
April 7	Avocado Chicken Salad	Avocado, chicken breasts, hard-boiled eggs, corn, flax seeds, lettuce, salad dressing	Some bloating	Sleepy	Fiber, PUFS, mild stress

*highlight ingredients in red to note PUFS content

Fig. 5: Use this log to track what you eat and how you feel afterward, helping you connect the dots between your diet and your overall well-being.

Earn a "Microbe Master" Badge

Are you ready to turn your gut health into a playful challenge? Let's talk about earning a "Microbe Master" badge. Sure, it might sound goofy, but this fun exercise can be a powerful motivator.

Here is how it works: Once you finish your Gut Health Quiz, set a simple goal for the week. It could be to replace two seed-oil snacks with alternatives made with butter or coconut oil. Another option is to try one new vegetable. As you knock out each goal, award yourself a mental "Microbe Master" badge.

If you want, feel free to take an old-school approach and place a medal or star sticker on your calendar to mark your triumphs. Alternatively, keep a digital scoreboard on your phone. The badge's purpose is to encourage positive habits and celebrate each small win along the way. Let's face it: We all like a pat on the back. That said, improving your gut health can feel like an invisible victory. People notice when you lose weight or change your hair color, but they rarely see the behind-the-scenes improvements associated with gut health. The badge reminds you that you're leveling up, even if no one else sees it.

If you really want to double down, recruit a friend or family member to join you. Challenge each other to see who can accumulate the most "Microbe Master" badges in a month. You may find yourself spontaneously sharing meal ideas or exchanging quick tips, such as which restaurants avoid seed oils and how to sneak more vegetables into a rushed weekday dinner. The sense of camaraderie can keep you from sliding back into old habits, especially on days when stress is high. Simply talking with an understanding buddy can ease your frustration and keep you from snacking on a not-so-gut-friendly treat.

The fun comes once you rack up a certain number of badges. That is when you can treat yourself to something that's not food-related, like a new pair of walking shoes or a cozy blanket. Every time you enjoy the item, you will remember that your achievements are all about caring for yourself. You are reshaping your gut environment in a lasting way.

Nurturing a Diverse Community: The Key Takeaway

Your gut is home to an incredibly varied set of microbes that work together to support digestion, immunity, and overall well-being. Nevertheless, these microbes can only do their job if you feed them the right substances. Seed oils brimming with PUFS can tip the balance toward inflammation-friendly strains, while a steady stream of fiber—once your gut health is balanced—encourages beneficial microbes that churn out Gut Gems.

So, remember, you're the one who decides what fuel you use for your microbial city each day. Sure, marketing and social pressures might push you toward choices that are high in PUFS, but your gut knows better. It's begging for nourishment that fosters balance and health from within. If you're willing to support it, your gut will return the favor in more ways than you imagined.

>————◄

Mara Meets Dr. Ellis

After dinner, Mara collapsed onto her plush couch. She folded her knees to her chest and clutched her stomach in pain. Mara groaned into the white pillow and stared sideways out the window to the dusk autumn streets of Chicago beyond. Leaves of orange and red dusted the urban street. It was her favorite time of year, and normally she would have plenty to do, but all she wanted was relief from her pain. She felt like she'd been hit in the gut with a baseball bat. She thought, *What on earth is happening to my body?*

She propped herself up and drank a glass of water, as if that would help. She pulled her dark hair back into a ponytail and fixed her hands on her hips. *I must be pushing myself too hard at the gym,* she thought. *Yes, that must be it. I'll feel better once I eat something.* Mara wandered into her kitchen and cooked her usual post-work-out meal: lean chicken and stir-fry vegetables sautéed in canola oil. She sampled a few savory pieces, and her gut seized in a spasm. *How can I have such a healthy diet yet feel so miserable?*

The next day, while driving in her car on her way to her niece's football game, another gut spasm flared in her gut. Her eyes watered. She had to pull over. *It's never been this bad before,* Mara thought, and she pulled out her phone. She booked a next-day appointment with Dr. Ellis, a no-nonsense functional medicine doctor recommended by her friend Sarah.

The following morning, she sat in Dr. Ellis's office and listened to the trickle of the indoor fountain. The windows were open, and a fresh breeze filled the room. Interesting. She had never felt so at ease in a doctor's office before. Outside, birds sang a trilling tune.

Dr. Ellis strode in with a big smile and an open demeanor. He was unlike other physicians who hurried through their patient list as quickly as possible. And he didn't probe her with questions about calorie counts or exercise regimens. He sat across from her for a while, reading her chart, with one foot balanced over his knee. He pushed his glasses up the bridge of his nose and said, "Your diet might be ruining your gut microbiome."

Mara tensed. She was a seasoned gym-goer, meticulous about labels and macronutrients—carbs, proteins, and fats. Was he suggesting she had done it wrong all these years?

But Dr. Ellis reassured her and explained the details of polyunsaturated fats and their influence on gut function, and Mara's curiosity sparked to life.

That night, as she lay in bed, she replayed Dr. Ellis's words in her mind. Maybe this was her chance to fix whatever was going on in her gut, or maybe it was just another false promise. She stared at the wood beams in the ceiling, and Dr. Ellis's warning rang in her ears: "You might think you're eating the right fats, but your gut microbes tell a different story." He was not a fan of canola oil, which Mara used all the time when she cooked. In fact, Dr. Ellis wasn't a fan of any oil that contained PUFS. But what did he know? Seed oils were a part of almost every health trend she'd tried over the past ten years.

Exhausted but unable to sleep, Mara wandered back into her kitchen. She snapped on a lamp and searched the labels on every box and bottle in her pantry. Her jaw dropped. Almost all of the packaged foods contained soybean oil or sunflower oil, which were on Dr. Ellis's no-go list of PUFS.

Mara couldn't help but wonder, *If I've been eating so many PUFS and feeling so awful, maybe there really is a connection.*

CHAPTER 2

Gut Gems—Your Gut's Secret Weapon

Your gut is an entire ecosystem that affects every aspect of your health. At the heart of your miraculous gut are Gut Gems, the short-chain fats your microbes churn out when they use fermentation to break down dietary fiber. By the way, if you're wondering, dietary fiber is the *indigestible* component of the plant-based complex carbohydrates you eat.

Gut Gems help reduce inflammation, fuel the cells that line your colon (called colonocytes), and influence your stress response. Seemingly miraculous, Gut Gems carry out basic biology. Give your gut the right ingredients and your microbes become a top-tier production crew, pumping out Gut Gems that your cells use to keep you well. Starve or stress your gut and the production line slows to a crawl, leaving you more vulnerable to health issues.

Unfortunately, modern living tends to disrupt the gut's daily operations. This chapter zeroes in on Gut Gems, exploring the nitty-gritty of how these tiny compounds power your entire system. We'll also see why certain microbes are crucial for cranking them out.

Inside the Microbial Gut Gem Workshop

Inside your gut, trillions of tiny microbes are working to break down various types of fiber. Among them, inulin is a natural fiber found in foods such as garlic, onions, bananas, and chicory root. Your body can't digest it, so inulin travels to your large intestine where helpful gut bacteria ferment it and convert it into Gut Gems.

How well your gut makes Gut Gems depends on things such as your gut pH (how acidic your gut is) and transit time (how quickly food moves through your digestive system). When everything is working correctly, Gut Gem production is strong. But modern habits—such as eating too little fiber, being stressed, or sitting too much—can throw off the process. That can lead to fewer Get Gems and more problems with digestion and overall health.

Three Super-Star Gut Gems

There are many different types of Gut Gems. We will focus on three of the most important: acetate, propionate, and butyrate.

Picture your gut like a workshop where microbes clock in and out, each with a unique specialty. Some excel at generating acetate, others crank out propionate, and still others produce butyrate. Together, Gut Gems form a behind-the-scenes power team that regulates everything from immune function to metabolism. If you're getting enough support from these compounds, your day might flow more smoothly, with fewer random aches, a steadier mood, and a noticeable sense of physical ease and internal balance. If your gut environment is unbalanced, maybe from repeated antibiotic use or constant exposure to PUFS from processed foods, the workshop grinds to a halt.

Acetate, propionate, and butyrate each have unique jobs, but they all revolve around helping gut cells thrive. Butyrate, for instance, keeps your colon lining well sealed, so unwanted particles can't slip through and trigger inflammatory responses. Propionate pitches in by influencing how your liver manages fructose metabolism, which can affect your energy levels throughout the day and whether you feel hungry soon after eating. Acetate moves more broadly, traveling around your system and sometimes even showing up as a fuel source for other tissues, such as muscles.

Gut Gems work together to create a stable, balanced state you can count on. The synergy, however, doesn't appear by magic. Certain microbes are real Gut Gem powerhouses, including *Faecalibacterium prausnitzii* and *Akkermansia muciniphila*, which helps pump out butyrate. (We will talk more about these microbes in the follow-up book, *Gut Cure 2*).

That said, these and other beneficial strains are easily undermined by toxins or an endless supply of junk food. If your gut is overrun with the wrong crowd of microbes, perhaps because you've been snacking on chips, the invaluable butyrate producers dwindle, leaving Gut Gem production in the gutter. What you need is a gut environment that supports the right microbial team—one that's ready, willing, and able to produce Gut Gems on a consistent basis.

Three Super-Star Gut Gems

Gut Gem	Made By (Gut Bacteria)	Where It's Made in the Gut	What It Does in the Body
Acetate	• *Bifidobacterium* • *Akkermansia* • *Prevotella*	Mostly in the first part of the colon	• Helps make fat and cholesterol • Can travel to the brain and help control appetite
Propionate	• *Bacteroides* • *Veillonella* • *Dialister*	Also in the first part of the colon	• Used by the liver to make sugar • May lower cholesterol • Helps you feel full
Butyrate	• *Faecalibacterium* • *Roseburia* • *Eubacterium*	Mostly in the last part of the colon	• Feeds the cells that line your colon • Lowers inflammation • Keeps your gut lining strong and healthy

Fig. 6: This quick glance at what these Gut Gems do shows just how important they are to whole-body health.

Why a Toxin-Damaged Gut Fails to Make Gut Gems

If you have been glancing at your snack stash and noticing everything is loaded with seed oils or other questionable ingredients, do not be shocked that your gut might be struggling to make Gut Gems. Toxins degrade microbial diversity. Without that variety, the synergy required to break down certain compounds and pump out Gut Gems does not happen. Instead, you are left with a fraction of the microbial workforce, which cannot keep up.

The issue is not merely about losing a few "good" microbes. The entire ecosystem can shift, favoring strains that thrive in a toxic environment over those that help produce Gut Gems. The less-helpful strains often churn out compounds that lead to inflammation or hamper digestion, creating a feedback loop of discomfort and gut issues. Meanwhile, you are trying to function on minimal Gut Gems, which can leave your cells starved of the nourishment and regulatory signals they count on.

The kicker is that once the downward spiral begins, it can be self-reinforcing. A gut bogged down by toxins tends to crave more processed foods—substances that keep the negative microbial cycle alive. As a result, you might crave refined fructose-filled pastries or PUFS-rich crunchy snacks, the very things that feed those gut-sabotaging microbes. Breaking that loop requires a willingness to kick old habits. Yes, this might mean ditching certain packaged items you may have grown to depend on. The payoff is a chance to restore your gut's capacity to make Gut Gems, which will allow you to reclaim that long-forgotten sense of well-being.

The Downward Spiral: How Toxins Impede Gut Gem Production

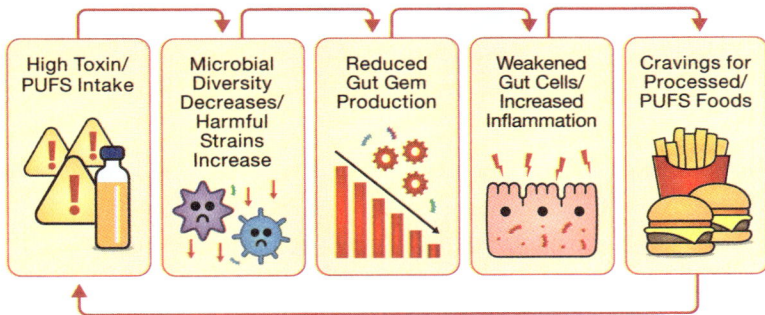

| High Toxin/ PUFS Intake | Microbial Diversity Decreases/ Harmful Strains Increase | Reduced Gut Gem Production | Weakened Gut Cells/ Increased Inflammation | Cravings for Processed/ PUFS Foods |

Fig. 7: Consuming foods that are laced with toxins sets off a chain reaction that impairs gut health and results in increased cravings for more harmful foods. Swapping out PUFS for healthier fats is a powerful way to interrupt the cycle.

Resistant Starch: A Powerful Ally—But Only When Your Gut Is Ready

If your gut is severely compromised, you may already be cautious about fiber—especially if it triggers immediate discomfort, such as bloating or cramping. Similarly, resistant starch deserves the same level of attention. While often promoted for its gut-healing potential, it can backfire if your gut is overwhelmed by harmful microbes or inflammation.

Resistant starch is technically a type of fiber, but it behaves a bit differently. It forms in foods such as rice and potatoes once they've been cooked and cooled—think leftover rice or chilled potato salad. When your gut is in good shape, resistant starch can act as a powerful ally, feeding beneficial microbes that slowly ferment it into Gut Gems. These compounds support the gut lining, regulate inflammation, and enhance microbial diversity.

However, just like other fibers, resistant starch can be hard to tolerate if your gut environment is out of balance. When harmful bacteria dominate, feeding them with resistant starch too soon may worsen symptoms like bloating, gas, and discomfort. The problem isn't the resistant starch itself but that your current gut population may not be equipped to handle it yet.

That's why a phased approach works best. First, reduce toxic inputs such as processed seed oils and other additives. Next, give your gut a chance to stabilize with meals centered on saturated fats, including butter or ghee. Other great options are foods that contain the odd-chain saturated fat C15:0. Along with whole-fat dairy products, good sources of C15:0 are fatty fish such as cod and sardines, as well as shellfish, beef, and lamb. For vegan alternatives, you may want to consider artichokes, asparagus, garlic, and onions. We will explore C15:0 further in chapter 19. For now, take pleasure in sampling and adding foods that appeal to your taste buds.

Once your digestion feels more settled and your symptoms have eased, you can test your tolerance for resistant starch. Start with a spoonful of cooled white rice or a few bites of potato salad. Observe how your body responds. Did you feel gassy, sluggish, or fine? If things went smoothly, you may gradually introduce more. However, while your gut is still in disarray, hold off. Let your system regain its footing before you introduce another task. Resistant starch can become a Gut Gem generator, but only when the timing is right.

Gut Gem Pop Quiz

Let's turn your growing Gut Gem knowledge into a friendly, low-pressure challenge. Each day, check in with yourself by asking two quick questions:

1. Did I avoid one PUFS-heavy food today?
2. Did I use a stable fat such as butter, ghee, coconut oil, or tallow in at least one meal?

Keep a simple daily log. Give yourself one point for each "yes" answer—up to two points per day. For example, did you skip the bag of seed oil–fried chips? That's one point. Did you cook your dinner in butter instead of using a store-bought sauce with canola oil? Another point for you!

Aim for a perfect score of fourteen points per week. If you land somewhere between ten and fourteen, you're building excellent momentum. Even seven points show a meaningful shift.

Set a milestone. If you reach twenty points within two weeks, reward yourself with something nonfood related—maybe the book you've been eyeing, a midweek movie night with a friend, or a small splurge that makes your space feel good.

As you keep track, you might notice changes: fewer cravings, smoother digestion, and a more even-keeled mood. The point isn't perfection; the purpose is to build awareness and momentum. Let the points be a tool that helps you tune in to your body's signals and celebrate progress without pressure.

Tying It All Together: The Future of Your Gut Gem Production

If you take away one crucial message from this chapter, let it be this: Gut Gems are your gut's internal glue. They help keep everything from your immune system to your mood in relative harmony. However, the glue holds only if you minimize daily toxins, especially PUFS-filled foods, while consuming the kinds of saturated fats that your gut can handle. If your gut is in crisis, you might avoid fibrous foods and those containing resistant starch. In the beginning, support your microbial metropolis by adding saturated fats and moving away from PUFS.

Later in the book, we'll talk about how to use carefully chosen probiotics to jump-start Gut Gem production. Just keep in mind that these are stepping stones to better gut health, not long-term solutions. The real fix is to create an environment where your Gut Gem producers flourish on their own. That means shifting your gut's equilibrium through mindful choices about what you eat, how often you rely on antibiotics, and how you handle daily stress.

As you move on to the next chapters, remember that everything from your daily routine to your cooking choices can either boost Gut Gem production or sideline it. So, stay curious, stay flexible, and remember that your gut is not a waste-disposal unit. It is a living system that can determine how you feel every day.

━━◄

Mara Doubts Her Diet

That morning at the gym in downtown Chicago, Mara felt unusually out of place. The clang of barbells and the hum of treadmills formed a familiar soundtrack that usually pumped her up. But today, it faded into the background. She lifted weights with her friend Jake, and usually they would chat with lively conversation, but she scowled at the floor between her tennis shoes.

"You seem kinda quiet today," Jake said.

"You know how I sometimes have those aches in my joints?"

"Yeah," Jake said, cautious.

"My doctor thinks my diet is the problem. He keeps talking nonsense about short-chained fatty acids." Mara huffed with each lift. "It's like I can't get Dr. Ellis's voice out of my head, you know? So many of my post-workout protein bars are technically a 'processed food' with 'PUFS,' but is that really so bad?"

"I eat them," Jake shrugged. "I don't cook."

Mara rolled her eyes, "I know, but why?" she groaned. "Why do I have joint aches if I've been eating this way for years?" She lifted thirty-pound barbells, one in each hand, and shot him an intense look. "Haven't I eaten all the recommended foods? Why would my diet suddenly be the problem?"

Mara retreated to the locker room after her workout and scarfed down a vanilla-flavored protein bar containing PUFS. It could be that it wasn't the best food choice, but who cared? She was ravenous. And besides, Dr. Ellis was too picky.

As Mara drove home, pain gripped her abdomen. She gasped for air. The pain twisted her gut and tears formed in her eyes. It couldn't have been the protein bar, could it? She curled into the steering wheel. *No,* she thought, *I've only been pushing myself too hard at the gym.*

That night she prepared her usual fried-chicken meal, but her hand hovered over the canola oil. She hesitated: "Maybe it wouldn't hurt to see if Dr. Ellis was right." She rummaged in the cabinet for some nearly forgotten coconut oil, and scooped it into the pan instead. It sizzled and the warm, nutty aroma surprised her. She took a bite, and she had to admit she loved the flavor and the crispiness. To her shock, she digested the coconut oil well. *Not bad,* she thought. *Not bad at all.*

><

CHAPTER 3

When Fiber Fails: A Postbiotic to Probiotic *Akkermansia* Ramp

We've already met the Gut Gems—the microbial MVPs that help restore order in your gut. But when it comes to true cellular renovation, one molecule deserves the spotlight: butyrate. If your gut were a renovation project, butyrate would be both the lead contractor and the power grid, rebuilding damaged infrastructure while keeping the lights on. It's not just helpful. It's foundational.

Your body can't make butyrate on its own. You've got to rely on your gut microbes to do the job, and only if you feed them the right kind of fiber will they pay you back with this powerhouse molecule.

Butyrate is produced when beneficial gut bacteria ferment specific kinds of fiber, namely resistant starches and prebiotic fibers found in foods such as green bananas, cold potatoes, and legumes. Not all fiber is equal, and not all bacteria know how to make butyrate. That makes this molecule a rare and valuable by-product—a metabolic reward for feeding the right microbes.

Among all the Gut Gems your gut microbes produce (including acetate and propionate), butyrate stands apart. It's the only one that fuels the very cells lining your colon—your colonocytes—providing up to 70 percent of their energy. That's like running your house almost entirely on solar power: clean, efficient, and self-sustaining.

But butyrate doesn't just provide energy. It feeds your gut cells in a way that helps them work faster and more efficiently than if they were running on sugar. It also tells your gut to tighten the seals between cells, patch holes in the lining, and rebuild the protective mucus layer that keeps harmful substances out.

On top of that, it quiets down the chemical signals that trigger inflammation. Using our house analogy, it rebuilds the broken plumbing, patches the leaky roof, and reinforces the front door. In short, butyrate is a real jack-of-all-trades and an incredibly helpful mechanic. Without it, your gut lining starts to crumble, those seals loosen, the protective coating thins out, and your immune system stays stuck in overdrive.

And the perks go far beyond digestion. When your gut is rich in butyrate, your inflammation levels drop, your immune response becomes more balanced, your mood lifts, and even your metabolism steadies. People often report fewer food reactions, better energy, and clearer thinking once they start producing more of this microbial gold.

So yes, butyrate is a big deal. In the pages ahead, you'll see how it works its magic and why making room for this VIP Gut Gem might just be one of the most powerful health upgrades you can give yourself.

Butyrate's Talent for Energizing Colonocytes

Let's dig further into what it means for butyrate to "energize" your gut cells. Your colonocytes are like miniature power plants in your colon wall. They need a steady fuel supply to repair damage, keep the gut barrier strong, and manage the constant traffic of nutrients and waste moving in and out of your intestinal lining. While they *can* run on glucose if they have to, that's like forcing them to burn firewood in a high-tech facility designed for clean energy. Butyrate is the premium-grade fuel they're built for.

Here's why: Butyrate slips directly into the mitochondria of colonocytes, where it's broken down through a process called beta-oxidation. This generates significantly more adenosine triphosphate (ATP)—the energy currency of your cells—than burning glucose does. If glucose is a backup generator that sputters along, butyrate is a high-efficiency solar grid that runs clean, cool, and powerful. Colonocytes thrive on it.

There's another reason butyrate fits the job so well. Your colon is a low-oxygen zone, which makes it hard for glucose to fully break down. But butyrate works beautifully in this low-oxygen environment. It's like having fuel that doesn't need much oxygen to burn cleanly and effectively—a rare find in the body.

This surge of efficient energy does more than just keep colonocytes alive. It gives them what they need to hold the line—literally. With enough butyrate, they maintain tight junctions (the seals between cells), replace damaged cells faster, and keep that protective barrier intact. When colonocytes run low on butyrate, they get sluggish, the gut lining weakens, and all sorts of unwelcome particles can breach the gut barrier. That is when you see problems such as food sensitivities, chronic bloating, and a host of issues that stretch far beyond the digestive tract.

It's easy to blame the usual suspects—stress, junk food, and certain medications—for causing gut misery. However, this misery also has fertile ground to grow if you do not have sufficient butyrate to feed your colonocytes. Think of a healthy gut as a fort surrounded by a sturdy rampart, whereas a leaky gut is more like an open pasture protected only by a makeshift crossbar fence.

Butyrate's Role in Inflammation

You might recall from a previous chapter that Gut Gems do an impressive job of lowering inflammation throughout your body. Butyrate is the main factor in that. It works like a chemical peacekeeper—stepping in when the gut is under attack and convincing your immune system to lower its weapons.

One of the ways butyrate does this is by calming a molecule called NF-κB (nuclear factor kappa-light-chain-enhancer of activated B cells; but don't worry—you won't be quizzed on it). Think of NF-κB as the fire alarm system inside your cells. It sounds the alarm any time there is stress or damage, which can be useful in short bursts. But if that alarm keeps blaring nonstop, your body stays in a constant state of inflammation. Butyrate walks in, pulls the batteries out of the overactive alarm, and tells your gut that the crisis is over.

Butyrate can also calm things down by talking to special receptors on gut cells and immune cells. It tells them to relax, and it even encourages the production of interleukin-10 (IL-10), a natural anti-inflammatory helper. It's like pressing a reset button for your gut's immune system.

It also quiets something called the NLRP3 inflammasome, which is like a cranky neighborhood-watch group that overreacts to every little disturbance. If NLRP3 stays hypervigilant, you end up with flare-ups of chronic inflammation not just in your gut but throughout your body. Butyrate helps it settle down, which can reduce inflammation markers such as C-reactive protein (CRP) and interleukin-6 (IL-6), both of which are often elevated in everything from arthritis to heart disease.

And speaking of real-world conditions, research shows that butyrate plays a role in improving symptoms of ulcerative colitis, calming joint inflammation in rheumatoid arthritis, and even reducing depressive symptoms, likely through its effects on inflammation in the brain. It's one of the few compounds that can influence the gut-brain axis by helping to regulate the vagus nerve, your body's main highway of communication between the gut and brain. It also helps quiet the brain's immune cells, called microglia, which get jumpy when inflammation is high.

One of the ways butyrate helps is by encouraging the growth of beneficial microbes, which in turn release other helpful compounds. At the same time, they crowd out the harmful microbes that thrive in inflamed environments. So, in a sense, butyrate gives your gut microbiome the tools to clean up the neighborhood.

You can think of your gut microbiome as a crowded neighborhood. Some neighbors are thoughtful, keeping their music down and helping you out when you need it. Others cause chaos, yelling in the street late at night, and throwing loud parties. Butyrate fosters a calm environment where the helpful microbes feel safe to thrive. When they do, they help keep things tidy, quiet, and inflammation-free, giving your entire body a break from the chaos.

Keeping Your Gut Lining Strong

We now know that colonocytes run on butyrate. If you imagine your gut lining as a fortress wall, your colonocytes are the bricks in that wall. Without enough butyrate, your colonocytes start running on sugar instead, which is much less efficient. That leads to a tired, worn-out gut lining, and the bricks start to crumble. Cracks form. Weak spots open. Soon, all sorts of undesirable particles begin slipping through the wall. The result is what many people refer to as a "leaky gut." In clinical terms, it's a loss of gut barrier integrity. When your gut barrier weakens, bits and pieces that should stay inside the colon sneak into your bloodstream. This can trigger a full-body immune response. That's why a leaky gut is now linked to conditions such as food allergies, eczema, autoimmune flare-ups, and even brain fog. What's more, one of the molecules that regulates gut permeability is called zonulin. When zonulin levels are too high, those tight junctions between cells loosen. Butyrate helps dial zonulin back down—like tightening the latches on your gut's protective gate.

But the barrier isn't made of just cells. Your gut is also protected by a two-layer mucus coating, and each layer has a job. The inner layer is dense and sticky, like a security screen. It blocks bacteria from reaching the gut wall. The outer layer is looser—home to friendly microbes that help break down fiber and produce more butyrate. When your gut bacteria aren't making enough butyrate, that inner layer thins out. Harmful microbes can then sneak past the screen and trigger inflammation. Butyrate helps rebuild both layers by feeding colonocytes directly and encouraging healthy microbes to repopulate the outer zone.

As if that weren't helpful enough, butyrate also flips on special genes that make proteins to tighten up the gut wall even more. And it blocks certain enzymes (called HDACs) that otherwise slow down repair work. Bonus twist? While butyrate serves as fuel in healthy colon cells, in colon cancer cells, it becomes a saboteur, blocking their growth and pushing them toward self-destruction. That's why high-fiber diets are strongly linked to lower rates of colon cancer.

So, to summarize, when colonocytes have a robust supply of energy, they replicate and maintain the gut barrier more effectively. That reduces the chance of a leaking gut barrier, causes fewer emergency flares of inflammation, and produces a generally healthier environment. It also means your body does not have to overreact to every morsel of food that comes through.

Do you ever have days when you feel like your body reacts to everything you eat? If so, your gut lining is possibly too weak, and when that barrier breaks down, even harmless foods can set off alarms. But you can fix this. With enough butyrate, your gut can focus on rebuilding, calming inflammation, and getting back to business.

How Butyrate Strengthens the Gut Barrier

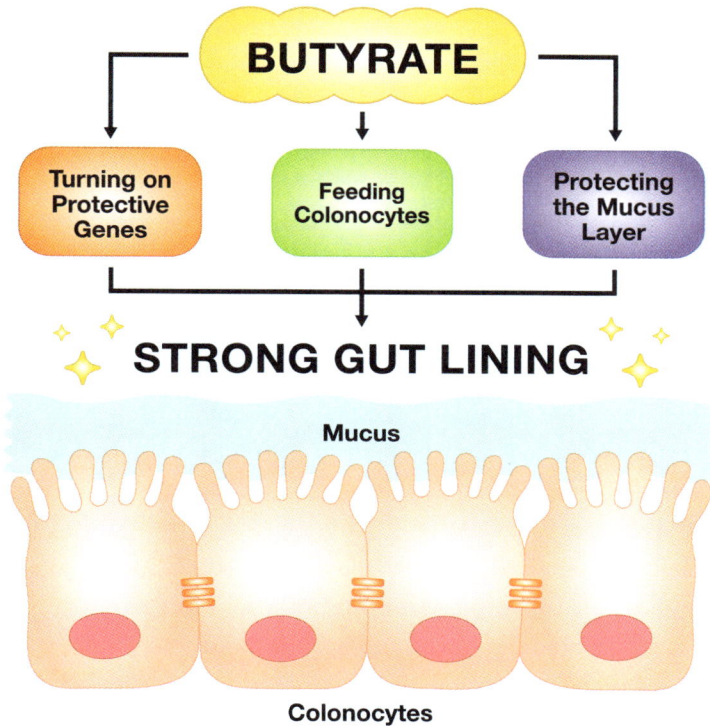

BUTYRATE

Turning on Protective Genes

Feeding Colonocytes

Protecting the Mucus Layer

STRONG GUT LINING

Mucus

Colonocytes

Fig. 8: Butyrate helps build a strong gut wall in multiple ways.

Butyrate for All-Over Health

What else happens when you maintain a butyrate-rich lifestyle? You might notice calmer moods; more resilient, less painful joints; steadier energy throughout the day; and a more consistent weight. That's because butyrate doesn't stop at your gut—it sends ripple effects throughout your entire body.

One major area it influences is the gut-brain axis. As mentioned, butyrate plays a starring role in this conversation. It helps regulate key neurotransmitters such as serotonin, which is involved in mood, appetite, and sleep regulation; and GABA, a calming brain chemical that acts like your internal "brakes," helping you relax and avoid anxiety spirals. Most of your serotonin is made in the gut, and it needs a healthy, low-inflammation environment to stay in balance. Butyrate helps provide exactly that.

Butyrate also protects your blood-brain barrier, a special filtering system that shields your brain from toxins and inflammatory molecules. When this barrier gets leaky, mental clarity, memory, and mood all take a hit. Butyrate helps tighten that barrier, reduce inflammation in the brain, and quiet overactive microglia, which are linked to depression when they're stuck in overdrive.

Then there's the metabolic benefit. Butyrate improves insulin sensitivity, which means your cells respond better to insulin and don't overstore fat after meals. That's a big win if you're dealing with blood sugar swings, stubborn weight, or energy crashes. It also helps regulate glucagon-like peptide-1 (GLP-1), the gut hormone that many new weight-loss drugs are designed to mimic. GLP-1 boosts satiety, improves blood sugar control, and supports weight loss—all things butyrate encourages naturally.

When you are not exhausted by blood sugar spikes or bogged down by chronic inflammation, your body has more bandwidth to do the things that matter. You can go for a walk, play with your dog, or tackle a big project at work without your brain constantly begging for caffeine or snacks.

And let us not forget that a well-fed gut also supports a balanced immune system, so you are not constantly fending off sniffles and strange aches. You experience clearer thinking, balanced emotions, and a sense that you can handle life's curveballs.

When you dial in a routine that supports butyrate production and reduces PUFS, you are effectively optimizing that gut-brain connection. You might notice you are less irritable, more creative, or simply content. These are not trivial perks. A calmer headspace can spill over into better relationships, improved work performance, and an all-around easier life. A contented gut can even lead to a happier outlook on life. Who doesn't want that?

When Fiber Fails: A Postbiotic to Prebiotic
Akkermansia Ramp

Your beneficial bacteria produce butyrate naturally when they feast on fiber. However, as explained earlier, a high-fiber diet can backfire if your gut is severely out of whack. That is the fiber paradox we talked about in chapter 1. When harmful microbes have taken over, adding more fermentable fiber is like throwing gas on a fire.

One workaround that can help you heal your gut without the discomfort of added fiber is to add foods that contain butyrate, such as butter. This is yet another reason to use it instead of seed oil. If you're dairy-free, ghee (clarified butter) will offer the same support without the casein or lactose. That said, butter or ghee alone will not give your gut all the butyrate it needs to rebuild.

The repair-first strategy I believe works best uses *Akkermansia*—beginning with a *postbiotic* form and progressing to a *probiotic* form once the lining has recovered. Postbiotics are not live microbes; they are the bioactive byproducts of microbial fermentation—such as Gut Gems, peptides, and cell wall components—that can directly support gut barrier repair and immune balance.

To begin the repair process, you first introduce postbiotic *Akkermansia*, which carries the membrane protein Amuc_1100. This step is crucial when fiber backfires, because it delivers "repair signals" to the mucosa without feeding a dysbiotic fire. Amuc_1100 is a tough, outer-membrane protein that sits on the surface of the bacterium. Think of it as a kind of antenna. When it comes in contact with the intestinal lining, it binds to a receptor called TLR2. That connection kicks off an anti-inflammatory signal that helps tighten up the "zippers" between intestinal cells. Those zippers—known as tight junctions—are the difference between a strong, selective gut barrier and a leaky one that lets harmful molecules seep into the bloodstream. In other words, Amuc_1100 is one of *Akkermansia*'s main tools for protecting the integrity of our gut wall. It helps accelerate epithelial repair and tight-junction support, giving the colon a chance to stabilize. The right delivery method is essential though. Naked proteins rarely survive the harsh environment of the GI tract, so they must be coated in something that allows them to reach their intended target (the colon). A postbiotic supplement's journey can be likened to a rough obstacle course. It starts in your stomach, where acid and pepsin go to work. Within the first hour, about 80 to 95 percent of a protein like Amuc_1100 is already broken down, leaving just 5 to 20 percent intact. Next stop is the small intestine, where even more digestive enzymes chip away at it, cutting that remainder by another 50 to 70 percent. By the time what's left reaches your colon, enzyme activity is much gentler—but at that point, there's usually only a tiny fraction still intact.

That is why successful programs use pasteurized whole *Akkermansia* or outer membrane vesicles, and protect them with an enteric coating or microencapsulation. Enteric coating is a protective layer added to supplements that keeps them from dissolving in the stomach's acidic environment. The coating is designed to stay intact until it encounters the higher pH or specific enzymes in your colon. Once it reaches the proper environment, the coating automatically dissolves and releases the active ingredient right where it's needed. Because this mechanism depends on your gut's natural chemistry, not the speed of your digestion, the release is personalized for every person. If a protected product isn't available, you can theoretically compensate with about 100 times the dose, but that's an inelegant, costly workaround. So, choose postbiotics with enteric coating or microencapsulation whenever possible.

After a few weeks to months—once symptoms quiet and the epithelium has at least partially healed—move on to the reseeding phase by gradually introducing *live* (probiotic) *Akkermansia* alongside gentle prebiotics your gut can tolerate. This is where the heavy lifting by butyrate and other Gut Gems like propionate and acetate, happens: oxygen-sensitive producers flourish again, and your own microbes—not a pill—drive the Gut Gem supply. Go low and slow with the prebiotics so you support the new colony without triggering bloat.

As repair signals do their job and Gut Gem production rebounds from within, most people notice a steadier gut, clearer skin, and fewer aches—the predictable ripple effect of a calmer, less inflamed mucosa.

Once your gut has sufficiently healed, you can explore how you tolerate small amounts of fiber again. In the meantime, let fiber take a backseat so you can focus on repairing the very cells that handle all that fiber in the first place.

It also helps to know your fiber types. Resistant starches (found in green bananas, cold potatoes, or cooked-and-cooled rice) are particularly good at feeding butyrate-producing bacteria. Fermentable fibers, like inulin and fructooligosaccharides (FOS)— found in foods like chicory root, onions, garlic, and asparagus— can be powerful but irritating if introduced too quickly. Insoluble fibers, like wheat bran, don't feed microbes as much. They add bulk but not butyrate.

Not sure if your approach is working? Watch for signs. If your bloating gets worse, your stool becomes erratic, or your skin breaks out, your gut may need more time. If instead you start noticing calmer digestion, steadier energy, and clearer thinking, it's a good sign your colonocytes are finally getting what they need.

For a step-by-step protocol—including microencapsulation criteria, day-by-day titration, and how to time the move from postbiotic to live *Akkermansia*—see Chapter 16.

Gut Check: Could You Be Low on Butyrate?

Use this quick checklist to find out if your colonocytes might be starving for fuel. Check all that apply:

Digestive Symptoms
☐ Frequent bloating, especially after meals
☐ Loose stools or sudden urgency
☐ Constipation or incomplete elimination
☐ Food sensitivities you didn't used to have
☐ Feeling worse after adding fiber to your diet

Skin and Immune Clues

- ☐ Eczema, rashes, or mystery breakouts
- ☐ Seasonal allergies or histamine intolerance
- ☐ Catching every cold that goes around
- ☐ Ongoing low-grade inflammation (high CRP, etcetera)

Mood and Energy Markers

- ☐ Brain fog or forgetfulness
- ☐ Feeling wired-but-tired, anxious, or low mood
- ☐ Energy crashes in the afternoon
- ☐ Trouble sleeping or feeling unrested in the morning

Metabolic Signals

- ☐ Cravings for sugar or caffeine
- ☐ Weight gain around the belly
- ☐ Blood sugar swings or prediabetes
- ☐ Insulin resistance or metabolic syndrome

Scoring

- **1–3 boxes checked:** You're probably doing okay, but there's still room to optimize.
- **4–7 boxes:** Your colonocytes are likely running low. A butyrate boost may help stabilize things.
- **8+ boxes:** You're showing classic signs of a gut wall under stress. It's time to start feeding your gut from the inside out.

Next Steps: How to Fuel Your Colonocytes

Pick one to three of these strategies to start with this week:

- Swap industrial seed oils for butyrate-rich butter or ghee in one meal per day.
- Cut back on PUFS, emulsifiers, and artificial sweeteners that can thin the mucus barrier and lower Gut Gem production.
- Try a two-day butyrate reset: Remove all added sugars and seed oils, and load up on bone broth, butter, and easily digestible whole foods.

- If you checked three boxes or fewer, add a small amount of resistant starch (like ½ cup of cold potatoes, cooked-and-cooled rice, or green banana) to your meals.

- If your gut reacts poorly to fiber, try an enteric coated postbiotic *Akkermansia* supplement at a low dose.

———

Mara Compares Herself to No-Good Health Influencers

Back at home, sitting in her Greystone townhouse in the Douglas neighborhood of Chicago, Mara scrolled through her phone while she sipped her morning coffee. Her Siamese cat, Imbie, purred on the bench beside her and rubbed up to her side. Mara chewed a breakfast bar while she scrolled, and an image of a Fabio-lookalike fitness influencer lit the screen, selling his latest protein bar, undoubtedly filled with PUFS.

"Pah-lease." Mara rolled her eyes and swiped away.

Another health guru appeared in his place, this time with excessive Botox and wearing a bikini.

"Why is everyone always showing off their stomach?" she snapped.

Little Imbie purred in reply.

Mara wilted over her coffee. The truth is, she'd probably spent more time in the gym than even these fitness wannabees! But because of her constant bloating, she'd never enjoyed the whole "washboard abs" concept.

Out of nowhere, a voice spoke from her phone, and it sounded familiar.

"I know that voice." She picked up her phone again, and Dr. Ellis, her functional medicine doctor, spoke with a completely different attitude. He discussed the importance of fiber for digestion and how to heal the gut microbiome. "It's a sign!" she told little Imbie. "That's my actual doctor! I know him!"

The "sign" sent Mara on a delightful spree. She spent the morning prep-cooking meals while listening to some of Dr. Ellis's interviews and diet tips. She set her phone next to her saucepan and listened while she stirred. His voice blared through the phone. Something he kept bringing up was butyrate. Apparently it soothed inflammation throughout the body. She imagined how it might ward off the bacterial intruders that stoked her bloating and cramps.

Mara changed her food preparation methods. She sautéed her veggies—more easily digestible spinach and button mushrooms—in butter. Butter contained butyrate, a win for her gut.

Mara pulled out a wooden ladle and took a sip of her vegetable concoction—savory, buttery, delicious. She fixed a hand on her hip. One step at a time, she was going to get her gut health back, no matter what it took.

><

CHAPTER 4

What Your Gut Was Built For—and Why Today's Diet Throws It Off Course

Picture a time before snack aisles, drive-through restaurants, and PUFS-filled industrial oils in our boxed, bottled, and bagged foods. Thousands of years ago, our ancestors roamed landscapes that brimmed with unprocessed meats, wild plants, and the occasional root or fruit. Fiber wasn't something they had to think about; it was simply part of the natural backdrop of how they ate. In fact, our ancestors typically consumed between 50 and 150 grams of fiber per day. Gut Gems likely flowed steadily from all that fiber. For most people today, a more realistic target is 25 to 35 grams.

Long ago, humans didn't need to understand what was happening inside their bodies to reap the benefits of having cells that thrived. For them, a deep synergy with nature and whole foods helped create a gut environment resilient enough to handle both feasts and fasts.

Over millennia, this natural pattern shaped our genetic blueprint. The gut adapted to expect consistent challenges—fibrous or otherwise—and developed a dynamic microbial community to respond. In the modern era, however, that primal design collides with an onslaught of processed foods, toxins, and strained lifestyle choices. The mismatch is as stark as a caveman scrolling social media on a smartphone.

Although we may not want to spend our days on a hunt to survive, our cells still crave that ancestral rhythm. Unfortunately, today's environment overwhelms them with PUFS and other disruptors. The result is widespread gut issues that many people now assume are a normal part of life—until they discover it doesn't have to be that way.

You may have glimpsed your gut's potential during a brief "reset" period. Perhaps you ate more whole foods or took a break from your usual routine. During that time, you may have noticed that your digestion was better and your mood steadier. Those small windows echoed what your ancestors enjoyed daily, minus the sabertooth threats. Their diet, while not an all-you-can-eat buffet, was high in fiber without the consistent barrage of modern toxins. That is the core lesson: Your gut is designed for a certain way of living. If you ignore it, you risk losing the synergy and vibrant energy it was designed to produce.

How We Lost Our Gut Edge

Fast-forward from our ancestor's world to the dawn of the industrial era. New-world factories churned out refined flour and novel oils. Populations gravitated to cities, away from farm-fresh produce and traditional fermented foods such as sauerkraut, kimchi, and yogurt. Fermentation not only made foods last longer but also produced friendly bacteria that enriched their gut microbiomes. Even those who remained in rural areas replaced much of their traditional diet with modern convenience foods. The era of mass production was great for improving food accessibility, but it also introduced radical shifts in what the gut had to process.

Around the 1800s, the researcher Michel Eugène Chevreul famously isolated butyric acid—a chemical that, unbeknownst to him, had fueled human health for ages. But such knowledge, unfortunately, did not always translate to wise dietary choices. As industrialization evolved, the public embraced cheap, shelf-stable foods that offered convenience and less spoilage. The catch was that many modern options harmed the gut microbiome.

Crowded out by competing strains, beneficial microbes lost their ability to produce short-chain fatty acids—what we call Gut Gems. Over time, their decline has contributed to what many now recognize as the modern "fiber famine." In today's world, the abundance of ancestral fiber is no longer part of the everyday diet, and our microbes are feeling the loss.

Some cultures clung to fermented foods and other microbe-friendly traditions that naturally supported the production of Gut Gems and overall gut health, but global food systems eventually streamlined into mass-produced uniformity. As the food system veered into industrial convenience, we lost more than pristine farmland and fresh air. We relinquished a connection to our ancestral diets as well as the microbes that supported so much of how humans acted, thought, and lived for generations.

Gut Gem: The Secret Fuel of Our Ancestors

Mainstream health gurus tend to champion carbs, proteins, or specific macros (the balance of fats, carbs, and proteins). In contrast, our ancestors naturally embraced a lifestyle that produced a healthy amount of Gut Gems. Frequent movement, whole foods with plenty of fiber, ample sun exposure, and minimal toxins gave beneficial microbes all they needed for that task.

Around 1966, the researcher Robert E. Hungate took a giant step in our understanding of Gut Gems. He demonstrated that bacteria in the gut could break down plant fibers and produce substances we now call SCFAs, including butyrate. His work revealed that these potent molecules weren't just random by-products; they were evidence of a powerful collaboration between food, microbes, and the human body. In essence, he helped uncover the existence and role of the microbiome.

Hungate's findings opened the door to a new wave of research. By the late twentieth century, scientists began exploring how fiber, when fermented by specific gut microbes, leads to the production of SCFAs. Interestingly, as studies deepened, one thing became clear: The relationship between fiber and gut health did not produce a one-size-fits-all prescription for optimum health.

That brings us back to the fiber paradox again. While many assume the fix is simply to load up on fiber, that strategy often backfires when your gut is overrun with harmful microbes or weakened by repeated antibiotic use. In that case, fiber might fuel the wrong populations. Until the core imbalance is addressed, your gut won't respond the way you want it to. Therefore, the reset begins by restoring microbial balance, often by reintroducing stable saturated fats and other ancestral habits that quietly rebuild the foundation.

Ancestral Diet Reflection

Modern life is drastically different from the way our ancestors lived. Consider, for instance, the foods you habitually turn to. If your morning starts with a processed cereal bar or a grab-and-go coffee drowned in PUFS-based creamers, that is a far cry from the nutrient-dense breakfasts of our forebears. They started and finished their days with whole foods. Frequently they would also skip meals.

Think, too, of how often you eat anything that's been fermented. How many times recently have you consumed beneficial gut microbes along with your food?

Next, think of your daily workload. Modern life often entails sitting at a desk for hours and maybe scrolling on your phone for entertainment. Your ancestors, in comparison, were constantly on the move. Fetching water, gathering wood, and chasing after animals were all part of life. Activity wasn't a half hour at the gym; it was baked into everyday living. Their constant movement not only kept them fit but also helped their gut process the foods they ate, facilitating Gut Gem production.

Now, think about your current lifestyle. Are you stressed and sedentary? Are you living on prepackaged meals that your ancient relatives would barely recognize as food?

Recreate the Ancestral Plate: A Gut-Health Dinner Challenge

Invite your friends or family to take part in a gut-friendly challenge inspired by ancestral eating—where fiber was abundant and industrial fats did not exist. The goal is to recreate a meal that echoes the nutrient-dense, fiber-rich traditions of the past.

Start by planning an ancestral-style meal. Choose whole foods that your great-great-grandparents would have recognized: roasted meats or wild-caught fish basted in stable fats like tallow or butter. Add fiber-rich vegetables that are easy to digest, such as carrots, turnips, or gently sautéed greens. If your gut is still healing, go easy on raw vegetables. Lightly cooked options are easier to tolerate.

Once your meal is ready, sit down without screens or distractions. Slow down and taste the food. Notice the richness of saturated fats and the absence of that greasy aftertaste left behind by industrial seed oils. Afterward, take a moment to reflect. Does your digestion feel more settled? Do you notice steadier energy or fewer cravings?

Check in with yourself the next morning. Are you waking up with a clearer head or feeling less desperate for food right away? These small shifts are signs your gut appreciates the fiber and fat balance you provided. Now, imagine if you ate this way regularly, how much better you might feel!

Modern Life Starves Your Cells

You might think you're doing everything right—eating clean, skipping the obvious junk—but despite best intentions, modern toxins have a way of slipping in through the cracks. You'll learn much more about this in the next two chapters. For now, just be aware that some foods that *seem* healthy, such as "lite" salad dressings and low-fat snacks, often rely on refined fructose to boost flavor. That energy bar labeled "natural" might be packed with PUFS and little else your body can use.

Another factor of the modern lifestyle is the demand for quick-and-cheap solutions. When pressed to save time or money, you may be tempted to lean on processed conveniences. Granted, such items can sit in your pantry for months, but they rarely help your gut. They usually come loaded with PUFS or empty starches. Even if you attempt to offset the negatives with a salad here or there, the sheer volume of daily toxins can overshadow good intentions. The usual consequence is a slow-burn meltdown of the gut ecosystem, which might result in frustrating weight gain, unpredictable digestion, or fluctuations in your mood that you cannot quite trace to a single cause.

And it's not just about what you eat. A stressful workday or too little movement can also take a toll on your gut, slowing down its ability to produce Gut Gems—the compounds that keep digestion smooth and inflammation in check.

Fortunately you don't have to abandon modern life and move to a homestead. Small steps—like choosing saturated fats over PUFS or gradually reducing your reliance on over-the-counter drugs—can create breathing room for your beneficial microbes. Over time, the space allows those microbes to rebuild, produce Gut Gems, and restore a baseline of health.

><

Mara Goes Back in Time

At home, resting in her bed, Mara could not get comfortable. She tossed in the dark, trying to alleviate a painful cramp in her gut. *This can't go on forever,* she thought. Mara sat up, reached for her phone, and a photo of her grandmother appeared, along with the text: *Ten Years Ago Today.*

Mara smiled.

In the photo, her grandma Nana stands beside a picnic she prepared at the local park. Nana holds Mara and balances herself with a wood cane.

A lump formed in Mara's throat. That trip to Philadelphia to see her grandmother was the last time she saw her. Nana had cooked for her every day. During that time, she ate mostly fresh foods, even homemade bread. Nana was something magical. All her foods were wonderful, too, and cooking was her love language. Mara's gut had felt calmer, with no painful stomach cramps. Her energy felt fine. She didn't have any mood swings with Nana. At the time, she'd chalked it up to the relaxation of Nana's presence, but perhaps it was her cooking that truly solved her gut problems during that time.

Images of her go-to protein bars surfaced to her mind: Those "vitamin-enriched" bars that had virtually no expiration date. The protein powders with sweeteners and additives she couldn't pronounce. But everyone else ate them. The vending machine at the gym was full of them. Still . . . They had a strange aftertaste that she always ignored.

Nana was strong and lively, even without all the powders and bars, and she seldom relied on packaged foods.

Mara smiled at the photo and memory of Nana and swiped off her phone. Even now, Nana was blessing her with wisdom.

><

CHAPTER 5

How Seed Oils and Toxins Damage Your Gut Microbiome

Why are PUFS so harmful to your gut health? There are two primary reasons: They promote the growth of harmful bacteria *and* contribute to inflammation.

You may wonder what exactly goes wrong when your microbial balance tips toward unfriendly strains. In a nutshell, your gut can transform into an echo chamber for low-grade inflammation. Rather than focusing on tasks like producing Gut Gems or shielding your immune system, certain microbes ramp up the release of signals that keep your body in a mild state of alarm. Think of what would happen if a neighborhood-watch group spent their time arguing with kids who cut across people's lawns instead of taking steps to prevent burglaries. If your gut is focused on the wrong tasks, you may feel fatigued, suffer joint aches, or feel on edge for reasons you cannot explain.

Inflammation tends to creep in gradually, so you slowly realize that your body is not bouncing back the way it used to. Small injuries or colds may linger, your mind gets foggy from time to time, and you may crave more caffeine or wonder if you need more vitamins. All the while, the real root cause can often be traced back to your gut microbiome.

It's a double-jeopardy situation: Inflammation shifts your gut population, shrinking beneficial strains such as *Roseburia* and *Fae-*

calibacterium—two big producers of Gut Gems—while boosting pathogens.

When helpful strains drop in numbers, you lose their calming influence on the immune system. The result? More inflammation.

This consistently inflamed environment can bleed into all sorts of areas, such as handling stress poorly or frequently having gut flare-ups after large meals. If your digestive system is already upset, and you keep feeding it PUFS-filled foods, your body will probably require more time to recover. You can break the cycle in two ways: limiting toxin intake and reintroducing stable fats that do not fuel inflammation. Once your body senses the hostility dying down, beneficial microbes can reemerge to produce Gut Gems that help keep your gut environment calm and collected.

Omega-6 Overload: The 20:1 Dilemma

Not all PUFS are the same. They fall into two main categories: omega-3s and omega-6s. Omega-3 fats—found in foods such as fatty fish and oysters—have anti-inflammatory properties that support brain, heart, and cellular health. Omega-6 fats, in comparison, tend to drive inflammation when consumed in excess. That's especially true for the omega-6 fats found in seed oils—namely, linoleic acid—which are often extracted using high heat and chemical solvents. This processing oxidizes the fats, creating unstable compounds that disrupt cell membranes and fuel inflammation.

Your goal isn't to eliminate all omega-6s but rather to restore balance. Experts estimate our ancestors consumed omega-6 and omega-3 fats in a roughly 1:1 ratio. Today, most people consume fifteen to twenty times more omega-6s than omega-3s—a dramatic shift with real consequences. This imbalance doesn't just affect your cells. It alters your gut environment, too, allowing harmful microbes to thrive more easily. By cutting back on industrial seed oils, making sure you get enough omega-3s, and choosing more stable, saturated fats, you give your body a chance to move back toward equilibrium.

The Omega Imbalance: Ancestral vs. Modern Diets

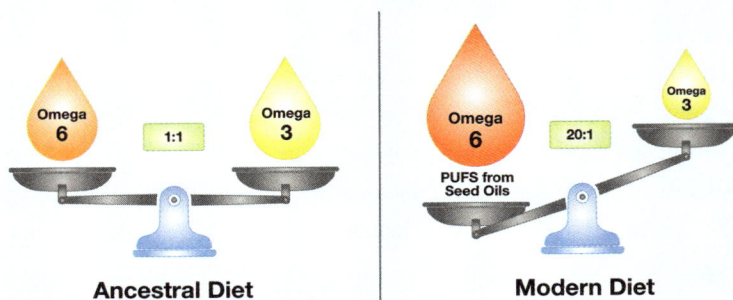

Fig. 9: Our reliance on PUFS (which contain omega-6 fats) creates a massive deviation from the omega-6:omega-3 ratio of our ancestral diet.

Processed Foods: A Double-Edged Sword

Processed foods are everywhere in our modern world. Convenience is king with vending machines tempting us at work, gas stations fueling our bellies on road trips, and the freezer section dominating the grocery store. Granted, time is valuable, but processed foods can contain an array of chemicals, synthetic sweeteners, and dyes that erode microbial diversity and promote the growth of unfriendly strains.

If you reach for a processed snack only occasionally, your gut can likely handle it without much trouble. Eating processed foods multiple times a day, however, will overwhelm your microbial metropolis and, over time, drastically lower Gut Gem production.

By replacing PUFS with stable fats such as butter, ghee, tallow, and coconut oil, you can reduce toxins that fuel harmful microbes and inflammation. Consistently using these preferred saturated fats will support beneficial microbial strains that produce Gut Gems, thereby stabilizing energy, curbing cravings, and combating the midday slump. Your gut is adaptable and can quickly pivot from a chaotic war zone to a thriving, well-coordinated community. Therefore, your role in this mission is to maintain consistency and avoid reverting to PUFS-filled foods that disrupt the microbial balance.

Fat Swap Challenge:
Discover Your Go-To Stable Fats

Objective: Reduce your PUFS exposure and discover satisfying, stable-fat alternatives you enjoy. This challenge helps you build new habits without feeling deprived—and shows your gut some love in the process.

Your mission: Swap out at least one PUFS-containing item per day with a saturated-fat-rich alternative.

How It Works

1. Pick a PUFS-rich food to replace: Scan your usual meals or snacks for seed oils, such as soybean, sunflower, safflower, canola, and "vegetable oil." Choose one that you'll swap today.

2. Choose a stable-fat alternative: Replace that item with a snack, cooking fat, or drink made from a stable, saturated fat such as butter, ghee, coconut oil, tallow, or full-fat dairy.

3. Track your swap: Use a notebook, app, or sticky note on your fridge. Each day you complete a swap, give yourself one point.

4. Earn bonus points (optional):
- +1 for trying a new stable-fat recipe
- +1 for reading a label and catching a hidden PUFS
- +2 for sharing a swap idea with a friend or online group
- +3 for preparing a meal using only stable fats

Food Swaps to Get You Started

- A square of high-quality dark chocolate (look for cocoa butter in the ingredient list, not a seed oil)
- Full-fat cheese with a few olives
- Toasted coconut chips or popcorn made with ghee
- Hard-boiled eggs with sea salt

Drinks

- Hot cocoa made with whole milk or coconut milk
- Coffee or tea with half-and-half or full-fat cream
- A small smoothie blended with coconut milk or grass-fed yogurt

Cooking Oils

- Use butter, ghee, tallow, coconut oil, or lard for roasting, sautéing, or baking
- Swap vegetable oil in a recipe with melted ghee or butter
- Fry eggs in butter or tallow instead of canola spray

When You Hit 30 Points, Choose Your Splurge

Splurge Option (Buy It): Pick up that one high-quality item you've been curious about—a block of aged cheese, a jar of grass-fed ghee, a kitchen gadget your friend swears by, or a grocery splurge that makes you feel taken care of.

Splurge Option (No Cost): Block out a few uninterrupted hours just for you. Cook a slow, satisfying meal. Sip something warm. Rest, read, or create. Give yourself the kind of day that tells your body you're worth the effort.

When Gut Gems Flow, Disease Retreats

Ultimately our focus is on PUFS because they disrupt the gut's ability to produce Gut Gems. Without adequate Gut Gems, your body loses a key line of defense against everything from random gut flare-ups to certain chronic conditions. Gut Gems tackle disease at its roots. They genuinely are that foundational. They keep your immune system from overreacting, help your gut barrier stay strong, and feed important cells that rely on these specialized fats.

Imagine waking up one morning feeling uncommonly light with sharper mental clarity and more control over your cravings. That describes the future that is possible when your body makes Gut Gems.

—◀

Mara Educates a Smoothie-Making Associate

As Mara pushed her cart through the aisles of her new favorite health food store in downtown Chicago, she spotted her favorite snack: kettle-cooked chips. The label on the bright-yellow bag of chips boasted "Low-Sodium and Gluten-Free." She grimaced and thought, *That may be true, but it still contains processed fats, and who knows what else.* Mara moved on and picked up a small tub of olives and a block of cheese instead.

If only I could eat these right now, she thought. Mara's stomach groaned. But eating olives in a store would be messy, and she had no fork.

The grocery store smoothie bar came into view and Mara beamed at it: "That's it." She shuffled up to it with her little cart and smiled at the high-school-age-looking guy behind the counter.

"I'll take a strawberry smoothie, please," she said. "All fruit."

"What?" the guy said.

"Strawberry," she said.

"A strawberry what?" the kid raked a hand through his tossed brown hair, and his eyes kind of floated around the grocery store.

"Smoothie," Mara said, short. "A strawberry smoothie."

"Oh, right on," the guy bobbed his head.

Mara's jaw tensed.

He took out his phone and looked at something.

"Well, are you going to make it or not?" Mara said.

"Ummm . . . yeah . . . yeah can do," he flipped his hair a little. "That'll be, like, fifteen minutes. Come back then."

"Aren't you going to ask me what size I want?" Mara pushed.

The guy puckered his lips and tilted his head a strange way. Slowly he asked, " . . . Size?"

"Large. Large is fine," Mara huffed, turned, and strode to the produce section.

Unbelievable, she thought. Mara sorted absently through the fruit, picking up odd apples and oranges for no particular reason. "Some people have children like that. They never teach them anything. Like manners. Like how to . . ." Mara stopped mid-step. She gripped an apple in her hand. She gently put it back.

She tilted her head, realizing she was hangry. Hungry and angry. Ha!

"My mood has gotten worse lately." She cracked a smile. "I should really work on that."

She took a deep breath and let it out. It was not the smoothie guy's fault he didn't know how to make a simple smoothie.

But when she returned to the smoothie stand, for some reason he looked surprised to see her. He patted around the counter until he found her smoothie and slid it across to her.

"Thanks," Mara said with a forced smile.

The guy bobbed his head.

Mara took a sip, sampling the flavors: Strawberry, yes, but a ton of sugar and something sour, something with the texture of sand.

Mara's eyes watered. "Woah, that's sweet. What's even in this? It was supposed to be all-fruit."

The guy flipped his hair and wiped his hands on his brown apron. "Yeah, that's the enhancer powder," he twitched and flipped his hair again. "It's, like, a powder we add. To enhance."

"I didn't ask for it," Mara said, pushing down the fire within. "Can I see the bottle?"

The guy handed over the tub with the powder he used. Mara flipped it over and read the ingredients list. One of the first ingredients: *grapeseed oil.*

"Ugh!" Mara said.

"What?" The guy panicked.

"You fed me something I can't eat. It's harmful to me. You can't just do this to people."

The guy flapped around. "I think it's a powder . . . I think it's okay . . ."

"You thought wrong. It's PUFS! You know what that is? An industrialized seed oil."

The guy stopped, then took her in with large, brown eyes. Then he chuckled a little: "I think you said a word, and . . . I'm not sure what that word means, but . . ."

"It means stop," Mara pushed the cold pink smoothie back to him over the counter. Her chest squeezed. Her breaths faltered. "These are bad smoothies."

A few passersby at the store noticed their feud and stopped to watch.

Mara's stomach dropped. She checked over her shoulder. People watched between the aisles. Had she really become that person who argues with a kid? Heat filled her cheeks. She swallowed hard and hurried out of the store.

Regardless, she had done the right thing. She had protected her health. Still, perhaps she had a ways to go. She still needed to work on her mood swings.

>————◄

CHAPTER 6

Find the Hidden PUFS in Your Diet

Once you start to look for PUFS on the ingredients list of the foods you eat every day, you'll start to see them everywhere. Strolling down a grocery aisle in search of a few convenient staples, you might pick up a box of cereal that boasts "heart-healthy" ingredients, a jar of peanut butter labeled "all-natural," and a package of whole wheat crackers promoted as a "smart snack." But when you flip over those packages and read the fine print, you're likely to find canola, soybean, or sunflower oil.

Is it possible that there are PUFS in nearly everything you eat? If most of your daily diet comes out of a box or a bag, the answer is yes. This is the harsh reality even if you've been taking care to select products you believe to be healthy.

Part of the reason PUFS have pervaded our food supply comes from the way the oils are marketed and pitched to the public. Packaged foods, as we've mentioned, might have a label that states it is "heart healthy." A big green checkmark or a leaf with words like "light" and "cholesterol-free" are also common. It all seems reassuring enough. But the chemical structure of the oils in these so-called healthy products tells a different story.

A hallmark of PUFS is that they are unstable, especially under heat. When exposed to high temperatures during cooking or processing, they break down and form harmful by-products such as aldehydes and lipid peroxides. Your body doesn't recognize these compounds, so it treats them like foreign invaders—sparking low-grade inflammation, disrupting your gut microbiome, and burdening your immune system. Over time, the internal stress they create can throw off your gut's delicate balance.

Why Most Labels Hide PUFS Behind Fancy Names

Ever read an ingredient list and feel like you need a translator? That is not an accident. Food manufacturers count on you glossing over complex or scientific-sounding terms. They highlight the buzzwords they know you're looking for—"organic," "non-GMO," "made with olive oil"—while the rest quietly hides in the fine print.

Take mayonnaise, for example. Brands such as Hellmann's and Best Foods market their classic versions as "real mayonnaise," made with "real, simple ingredients." Flip the jar over, though, and the first ingredient is usually soybean oil. Yes, eggs and vinegar are present, but the primary ingredient, a refined seed oil, is high in PUFS.

Olive oil–based mayo is also commonly deceiving. Many popular "olive oil mayonnaise" products still list soybean or canola oil as the main fat. Olive oil is added in small amounts—just enough to make the claim legally valid and catch your eye on the shelf.

You'll find similar tactics in packaged snacks. A bag of crackers might tout "baked, not fried," as if that automatically means healthy. But baked with what? Often it's canola, corn, or sunflower oil—seed oils used for texture and shelf life. The front may shout "whole grains," but the back quietly includes the very oils your gut may struggle to handle.

Cost is part of the equation. Seed oils are cheap—far less expensive than butter or coconut oil. That's why they show up in everything from cookies to cereals, snack bars to spreads. Peanut butter is among the worst. It already contains some PUFS by nature and often has added soybean or sunflower oil to stay creamy and shelf stable.

And don't be fooled by the word *natural*. A product labeled "natural" or "made with natural oils" can still contain highly refined industrial fats. By the end of the day, you may have unknowingly consumed a heavy dose of PUFS, all while thinking you were making smart choices. The fix? Don't stop at the front label. Flip the package over. Scan the list of ingredients. Remember, when it comes to protecting your gut and reducing inflammation, the real answers are always in the fine print.

Hidden PUFS Label Decoder

Not every label spells things out as clearly as "canola oil." Ingredients such as tocopherols (a form of vitamin E) or emulsifiers may not directly indicate the presence of seed oils. However, they can be part of processed blends that rely on them. Some manufacturers also get creative with how they present their fats. For example, "high oleic sunflower oil" might sound like a healthy upgrade, and it *is* more stable than standard sunflower oil. But it's still a refined seed oil that undergoes industrial processing that degrades its structure and nutritional value.

Other terms such as "expeller-pressed" may suggest a gentler extraction method, but that doesn't change the nature of the oil itself. Whether expeller-pressed or chemically extracted, canola, soybean, and sunflower oils remain high in PUFS with significant potential for oxidation—especially under heat. They are also high in omega-6 fats and can throw off your omega-6: omega-3 ratio, as mentioned in the previous chapter.

One major red flag to look for: "hydrogenated" or "partially hydrogenated" oils. These terms indicate the presence of trans fats, which have been linked to inflammation, heart disease, and other serious health issues. While trans fats are banned or restricted in many countries, they can still show up in small amounts in older products, certain processed foods, and imported items. If you spot "hydrogenated" or "partially hydrogenated" on the label, it's best to put that item back on the shelf.

Sweet treats are another hidden source of seed oils. Mass-marketed cookies, pastries, donuts, and candy bars often contain soybean or cottonseed oil to keep products shelf stable and inexpensive. If you're craving something sweet, you're better off baking at home with butter or coconut oil—fats that hold their structure and flavor under heat and let you control the ingredients.

Labels claiming "70% less fat" may sound like a win, but always check the ingredients list. If you see canola, soybean, or corn oil, you're still getting more inflammation than nourishment.

How Outsourced Meals Feed the Fire

Restaurants do not usually cook with premium animal fats or extra-virgin olive oil. Instead, they rely on seed oils, which are cheap, shelf stable, and neutral in flavor. Even when you order something that sounds "healthy," such as grilled fish or sautéed vegetables, it's likely cooked on a flat-top grill coated in soybean oil or tossed in canola oil before hitting the pan.

Your best move at a restaurant is to choose dishes that are less likely to be cooked or soaked in oil. A plain grilled steak or burger patty—with no marinade or added sauce—is a safer bet. Ask your server what kind of oil the kitchen uses for cooking. Is it possible to prepare your meal without the oil or with real butter instead? Not every restaurant will accommodate, but many will if you ask. Every small change can reduce your exposure to the worst offenders.

Social events such as dinner parties and family gatherings can pose the same challenge. Aunt Linda's famous casserole might be made with canned soup that contains soybean oil and pre-shredded cheese coated in anti-caking agents suspended in seed oils. If you don't want to dissect every dish on the table, stick to the simplest items. Go for the roasted meat, hard cheeses, and raw vegetables without dressing. You can also bring a dish of your own, giving you at least one safe option.

With time and awareness, you'll start to spot seed-oil traps before they hit your plate. The goal isn't perfection—it's progress. Each choice to limit PUFS exposure moves your gut one step closer to balance.

What About Nuts and Seeds?

Nuts and seeds are tricky. On one hand, whole foods such as almonds, peanuts, cashews, and pumpkin seeds can provide valuable nutrients. On the other hand, they contain a fair share of PUFS in their raw state, so eating them in large quantities could lead to an overload. This is particularly true for walnuts and sunflower seeds. Moderation is key. A small portion now and then is not going to undermine your health. But if you are eating handfuls of trail mix every day, you could be taking in more PUFS than you realize.

You may want to put nuts and seeds on pause entirely if you're in the early stages of lowering your PUFS load. Once you've stayed on a reduced-PUFS diet for a while, you can gradually bring back moderate portions of nuts and seeds.

Another hidden trap is nuts or seeds roasted in seed oil. You may see something such as "roasted in peanut oil" on a bag of peanuts. Another common sighting is flavored almonds that list canola or soybean oil as a "seasoning ingredient." If you're trying to be mindful, look for dry-roasted nuts with minimal additives or consider raw versions. Alternatively, you could lightly toast them yourself in a pan with a dab of coconut oil or butter. And don't forget the infamous nut butters. Peanut butter, almond butter, and so forth often have a bit of added oil to achieve their smooth texture. Soybean oil or canola oil are common in the cheaper brands. Likewise, expensive "natural" brands may slip in some seed oil to keep it from separating. Reading the label is your best bet. Ideally choose something that lists the nut itself and maybe salt. A brand that uses a safer fat will usually say so prominently as a selling point. Paying a little more for a quality product could be worth it.

Tackling the Great Snack Attack

Snacking is where many of us fall off the wagon. You can eat a pristine breakfast and lunch, but if you are starving at 3:00 p.m., that bag of chips from the vending machine can make you forget all the warnings about PUFS. The makers of chips, crackers, processed baked goods, and "healthy" fruit bars often rely on seed oils for shelf stability. Over time, your habitual snack can translate into a daily burden on your gut.

Instead, snack on fresh fruit, cheese (assuming it is made with animal rennet, not one that is synthetic and genetically modified), or an easy-to-prepare homemade treat. If you absolutely need something crunchy, look for items specifically labeled "fried in coconut oil" or "made with butter." They do exist, though you might have to search online or shop at specialty stores. Another approach is to make your own chips using thinly sliced vegetables or fruits. Brush the slices with butter or coconut oil, then bake until crispy.

Last but not least, check your beverage choices. Certain "nutritional shakes" and "coffee creamers" carry a surprising amount of seed oil in the form of emulsifiers. Switch to real cream if you handle dairy well or a coconut-based creamer that does not contain added seed oils. Or take the old-fashioned route: drink black coffee or tea without any additives.

Bridging the Gap When Others Aren't on Board

Having friends or family who are not on board can be challenging, especially if you often share meals. You have a few options. One is to educate them in a gentle way about your objectives. Show them the listed ingredients or talk about the difference in how you feel when you cut back on PUFS.

Another approach is to compromise. For instance, take charge of cooking the main meal a couple of nights a week. That way you can control the ingredients used. When you are not the one preparing for the group, you may need to keep your own stash of butter in a separate part of the fridge or have your own snack box on hand. The goal is not to force anyone else to follow your plan. At the same time, don't let others' choices sabotage your progress.

Overcoming the Fear of Saturated Fats

Many folks fear that switching from seed oils to saturated fats will sabotage their heart health. After all, the public was told for years that saturated fats were a recipe for an early death. Supposedly they clogged arteries, raised cholesterol, and led to heart attacks. Decades of research have challenged that old narrative.

If you are concerned about your cholesterol, consider doing your own research. Experiment with your own labs. Some people have their cholesterol and inflammatory markers checked before changing their diet and then test them again a few months later. They are often surprised to see improvements in overall markers, even if their total cholesterol shifts. Of course, everybody is different, and if you have a specific medical condition, you should keep your doctor in the loop. That said, do not allow the fear of saturated fats, fueled by misleading marketing campaigns, to prevent you from removing the more harmful seed oils that are quietly setting your gut on fire.

Once you've cleared the worst offenders, it's time to reintroduce fats your body actually knows how to use. Take coconut oil, for example. It's rich in medium-chain triglycerides (MCTs), which your body metabolizes more efficiently than the long-chain fats found in most seed oils. For many people, that means a more stable energy supply. Butter, in turn, offers a unique mix of nutrients—providing butyrate, fat-soluble vitamins, and conjugated linoleic acid (CLA)—you won't find in margarine. This is especially true when the dairy cow was grass-fed. These once-vilified fats could end up being the very key to unlocking a healthier, more resilient gut.

Pantry-Purge Mission: Take Your PUFS Detox a Step Further

The best approach in eradicating PUFS from your pantry is to identify where the biggest offenders are sneaking in. Is it that daily drizzle of cheap cooking oil in your frying pan at breakfast? Could it be that tub of margarine you reflexively grabbed because you have heard the "low cholesterol" hype for years? You know your habits better than anyone else, so zero in on the items that have caused you to consume seed oils without realizing it.

Perhaps the most straightforward first step is to swap out your cooking oil. Instead of using vegetable oil, cook with butter, coconut oil, tallow, or ghee. You might have seen a swirl of negative press about saturated fats, but keep in mind that a lot of that chatter originated from outdated science and marketing campaigns.

Second, if you love spreads and toppings, take a closer look at them. Are you using margarine or something from a tub labeled "spread" on your toast? "Spread" is typically code for "seed-oil mixture" with additives to mimic the taste and texture of butter. Next time, just purchase real butter. Ghee is a good option if you're sensitive to dairy proteins or lactose. It's a form of clarified butter, meaning most of the milk solids—including casein and lactose—have been removed during the clarification process. What remains is a rich, stable fat that tolerates higher cooking temperatures and is easier on digestion for many people with dairy sensitivities.

Finally, watch out for dressings, marinades, and sauces. They are often riddled with PUFS. If you can't find a butter- or coconut-based brand, try whipping up your own. Something as simple as melted butter with a dash of lemon juice, herbs, and salt can do wonders as a marinade.

One unexpected benefit of removing PUFS is the opportunity to explore more creative, tastier ways to cook. Experiment with different forms of butter-based sauces or coconut-oil stir-fries. You may discover that browning your veggies in butter creates a richer, more indulgent flavor than you ever got from vegetable oil.

Going on a culinary adventure can also reenergize your mealtime routine. You may read recipes that rely on stable fats or adapt old favorites with your new approach. For instance, try roasting potatoes in butter and rosemary or try lightly frying fish in coconut oil with garlic and herbs. Over time, you will develop a pleasing roster of go-to meals that fit your new mindset.

Envisioning a Life with Minimal PUFS

Imagine waking up in the morning, frying eggs in a pan with a bit of butter, and savoring the wholesome aroma. Maybe you top it off with a side of crispy bacon. At lunch, you drizzle your salad with a homemade dressing that took all of five minutes to mix. Dinner might be a steak with roasted vegetables on the side. For dessert, savor some homemade fudge made with coconut oil, cocoa powder, and maple syrup—an easy recipe that melts in your mouth and skips the industrial fats entirely.

Social events are more about what you bring to the table. Maybe you show up at a potluck with a butter-based casserole or a coconut-oil-based dessert. You may even convert a skeptic or two when they realize your dish is not only tasty but incredibly healthy. Also, maintain a rotating library of favorite recipes to avoid boredom. Experiment with new seasonings and cooking techniques. Connect with communities online or locally to swap ideas and stay motivated.

Your taste buds and cravings will usually shift once you make dietary changes, making the process all the more painless. You might think you'll miss your favorite PUFS-filled chips forever, but people often report that such cravings vanish after a while. Later, when they sample the old favorite again, many notice a chemical or stale aftertaste that was not obvious before. Your body will adapt to a new palate that prefers saturated fats, which taste better. At that point, steering clear of temptations becomes less about discipline and more about preference.

Going All In: Is Zero PUFS Possible?

By now you may think you should banish every trace of PUFS from your meals. But let's be honest: Aiming for absolute zero is practically impossible. In fact, many natural, unprocessed foods contain PUFS—for a good reason. Cells need around a gram or two of PUFS per day. If you are diligent, such as by sticking to butter and coconut oil, a small amount will slip into your diet through nuts, seeds, and other natural foods. The problem is that most people eat ten or twenty times that amount, and that's when trouble starts brewing.

A single meal will not necessarily set off the alarm, but the drip, drip, drip of seed oils in your coffee creamer, salad dressing, marinated chicken, snack bar, and bag of chips certainly will. Before you know it, your body is drowning in a sea of unwanted compounds.

The goal is to dial down your daily total to a level that keeps your gut calm—ideally under 5 grams a day or as low as 2 grams if possible. That's all your body needs, and it's very close to what our ancestors got from a whole food diet.

If you're scratching your head about how to measure your consumption, you can use the Mercola Health Coach app to see where you stand. This app will let you describe exactly what you're eating and show you down to the gram just how many PUFS are on your plate.

Scan this QR code to get FREE access to the Mercola Health Coach app. This tool allows you to log your meals, track your macronutrient ratios, and monitor your progress over time.

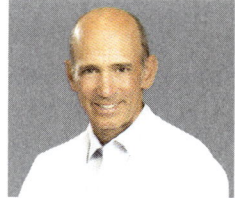

Mara Purges Her Kitchen

At night, Mara roamed through her home and reached into her fridge for her usual spoonful of peanut butter as her midnight snack. Her old staple would not let her down—after all, it was just peanuts. But she paused at the fridge. She had not examined its label when looking through her other pantry items. A nagging feeling made her flip the jar, and she saw it: *hydrogenated soybean oil.* Her chest sank and she put the jar down. Mara flipped on the lights in her bright, modern-style kitchen. She couldn't sleep anyway. This would be a night of momentous change. Tonight was the night she crossed the point of no return—she would eliminate everything, no more seed oils, no more PUFS. Dr. Ellis's words echoed in her mind: *You might need to check all the common foods in your pantry, and see what you really want to keep and what you shouldn't have as an option in the first place.*

Mara slid open the pantry and pulled jars from the shelves. Label after label revealed ingredients she had never questioned before. Granola bars claimed to be "heart healthy" but listed soybean oil. Her go-to cooking spray was canola oil, front and center. She ran a finger over the almost-empty bottle. How could she have trusted it? She tossed it away. Once, she had scoffed at butter, convinced by magazine ads that it was dangerous. A pang of regret hit her chest: "What else have I believed that wasn't true?"

Mara noticed the "low-fat" mayonnaise she frequently used on sandwiches. The bloating she blamed on stress now had a new suspect. She picked up the jar, turned it over, and read the label. Soybean oil. *Again! It's everywhere!* she thought.

Mara spent the night purging her kitchen. Once she was done, she felt lighter somehow. She was certain she could choose anything in her kitchen at all and make the right choice.

><

CHAPTER 7

Other Industrial Toxins— Why They Matter

You might be laser-focused on kicking out PUFS-laced products from your pantry, but a whole swarm of other industrial toxins are lurking in your food, eager to tag along for the ride. The culprits are emulsifiers that promise to make your sauces creamy, pesticide residues that upend your gut's balance, and preservatives that create infinite shelf life at the expense of your colonocytes. The subtle toxins can compound the damage to your gut if it is already wrestling with a PUFS-filled diet, leaving you in a tug-of-war between feeling less than okay and just plain horrible.

It might sound dramatic to label everyday ingredients as toxins, but they can inflict serious trouble. When your gut tries to handle a parade of additives and contaminants, your colonocytes get overwhelmed. They thrive on a calm, stable environment that fosters Gut Gem production and healthy hormone signals. Tossing in a host of preservatives and pesticide residue adds more roadblocks to an already jammed highway. You can imagine the domino effect that results when your colonocytes do not get the Gut Gems they depend on and beneficial bacteria lose their foothold. Your microbiome then changes for the worse.

Where Emulsifiers and Preservatives Hide

Food companies love to tell you they have made your life easier: Just add water for instant sauces, pop open a can of soup, and tear open a packet for a premixed marinade. The black magic behind many "convenience" items begins with emulsifiers and preservatives that promise to keep foods stable, sauces cohesive, and shelf life nearly immortal. The chemicals, however, can zero in on the gut's protective mucus layers and poke holes where none should exist.

Imagine your mucus layers as a fortress wall that stands between your colonocytes and whatever you just ate. Emulsifiers erode that wall, letting irritants agitate the colonocytes. Over time, the assaults stoke inflammation, hamper your gut's ability to produce Gut Gems, and weaken the beneficial bacteria that keep your hormones balanced. As for preservatives, they do a great job of keeping snacks edible for an eternity, but they act like speed bumps for your microbiome. While preservatives are terrific for preventing mold in your fridge, they disrupt the microbial balance in your gut if you pile them on daily.

Munching on preservatives day in and day out, especially on top of a diet high in PUFS, slowly chips away at your gut's resilience until you are more prone to discomfort, bloating, and a general sense of unease. Next thing you know, your beneficial bacteria are lagging, your Gut Gem supply is down, and you are toying with quick fixes to salvage your energy or control your weight. You can blame it all on ingredients you never realized were disrupting your gut behind the scenes.

When Pesticides Sneak In

Think about the last time you grabbed fresh produce from the grocery store. You likely assumed your choices were full of vitamins and minerals. They may also have sported a fresh coat of pesticides. Certain chemicals help farmers grow bigger, prettier crops, but your colonocytes pay a steep price. Glyphosate (Roundup), for instance, has a special knack for taking out beneficial bacteria right alongside the pests it is supposed to target. And while washing produce can help remove some residue, it doesn't remove systemic pesticides, which are absorbed into the plant's tissues as it grows. So, while you enjoy that crisp lettuce, your gut's friendly microbes might be suffering.

You might not notice an immediate meltdown, but over time, your gut environment becomes less diverse, less capable of pumping out Gut Gems, and less forgiving of occasional dietary slipups. Your colonocytes, in turn, might have to work overtime just to maintain normal function, and the effects can ripple through everything from hormone balance to your daily mood.

Switching to produce labeled "organic" can go a long way toward minimizing your pesticide exposure, but they're not always available or affordable. The best approach is to do what you can. Make sure you wash your vegetables thoroughly, look for local sources that rely less on heavy chemicals, and buy organic when you can. Every small step to lower the pesticide load can free up your gut to focus on Gut Gem production.

Plastics and Endocrine Disruption

If you are microwaving leftovers in cheap plastic containers or sipping water from an old bottle that leaches toxic chemicals, you could be giving your gut more to handle than you realize. Many plastics contain endocrine disruptors that confuse your hormone signals as well as your gut's microbial metabolism.

A stressed microbial community means fewer Gut Gems, and lower levels of Gut Gems mean your colonocytes will struggle to maintain normal hormone cycles. It is all interconnected, and exposure to endocrine-disrupting chemicals from plastics can throw everything out of sync. Imagine how toxins affect thousands of people, day after day. They brew coffee in a plastic machine that has seen better days. They eat meals from plastic containers that release trace chemicals each time they are reheated. Over time, every little exposure adds up, reinforcing a stressed environment that is already dealing with the damage from PUFS-filled oils and pesticide residues.

If you wrestle with energy crashes or mood swings, your system might be dealing with a chemical onslaught that is overshadowing all your best efforts to keep your weight and appetite stable. Swapping plastic for glass or stainless steel may seem like a small change, but it can go a long way toward protecting your gut from unwanted chemical assaults.

Identify Your Toxins

Reading labels can have a learning curve. If you are in your kitchen, rummaging through cupboards with a detective's eye and scanning labels for obscure ingredients such as emulsifiers, your actions may feel a bit extreme. But the payoff is huge once you start connecting the dots between a suspicious "emulsifier" in your favorite sauce and the achy stomach you experience two hours later.

As you read labels, keep an eye out for words like *carrageenan*, *polysorbate* (60 or 80), *monoglycerides*, *diglycerides*, and anything suspiciously ending in *-ate*. The complex names basically mean "industrial glue" that holds water and fats together in your food. They can also undermine that protective mucus layer in your gut. If you see a list of complicated terms you cannot pronounce—particularly in products promising extra-creamy texture or shelf-stable convenience—odds are you're dealing with emulsifiers that strip your gut lining of the protective barrier that keeps you feeling balanced.

As you weed out emulsifiers, preservatives, pesticides, and plastics from your food, pay attention to how you feel. Maybe you notice less bloating and a calmer state of mind. Over time, your new dietary choices could spare you from needing your monthly prescription or the next so-called miracle shot. Once your gut is no longer under a daily chemical assault, you can let it do its job: produce Gut Gems, balance hormones, and keep your hunger in line, all on its own.

Toxin Detective: Your Gut Health Mission

Let's make lessening your toxic exposures more fun by playing a little game. You're the detective, and your job is to track down and remove everyday toxins that may be messing with your gut. For every toxin you spot and swap, you earn points and bring your gut one step closer to balance.

How to Play

For each action you take, give yourself 1 point. Add up your score at the end to see how far you've come.

- **Plastic Containers:** Plastics can leach harmful chemicals into your food, especially when heated.

Give yourself 1 point for each action:

You swapped plastic containers for glass or stainless steel.

You avoided microwaving food in plastic.

You used a reusable water bottle that isn't plastic.

Points: _____ / 3

- **Pesticides:** Residue from pesticides on produce can disrupt the helpful bacteria in your gut.

Give yourself 1 point for each action:

You washed all fruits and vegetables thoroughly.

You chose organic produce.

You started to grow at least one of your own herbs or vegetables.

Points: _____ / 3

- **Emulsifiers:** Common in processed foods, emulsifiers can irritate the gut lining and affect gut bacteria.

Give yourself 1 point for each action:

You started checking ingredient labels for emulsifiers like polysorbate 80 or carboxymethylcellulose.

You reduced your intake of processed and packaged foods.

You replaced a processed item with a homemade version this week.

Points: _____ / 3

- **Preservatives:** Preservatives can help food last longer, but some may interfere with gut health.

Give yourself 1 point for each action:

You read labels and try to avoid preservatives like sodium benzoate, BHT, or nitrates.

You chose fresh or frozen foods over shelf-stable packaged ones.

You tried a preservative-free alternative to a food you usually buy.

Points: _____ / 3

Your Score: Total points: _____ / 12

0–4 points: Getting Started

You've begun the journey. Small steps lead to big changes.

5–8 points: Making Progress
Your gut is noticing the difference. Keep it up.

9–12 points: Gut-Health Hero
You're taking charge and making smart, sustainable choices.

The Domino Effect—Fewer Gut Gems, More Trouble

When your gut is hammered by emulsifiers, preservatives, pesticides, and endocrine disruptors, each behaves like a domino that falls onto the next one. Emulsifiers peel away protective mucus layers, pesticides mow down beneficial microbes, and endocrine disruptors from plastics can interfere with your hormone signals.

Add a diet already heavy with PUFS, and you have a perfect storm. Your colonocytes, battered by chemicals, cannot produce enough Gut Gems. Your microbes, under siege from daily toxins, cannot maintain a strong population. The deficiency in Gut Gems means a shortfall in how your body naturally regulates hunger and inflammation. You might be ravenous for no reason or notice that a small indulgence leads to bloating and extra pounds.

Recognizing the domino effect is half the battle. When you see how toxins work in tandem to degrade your gut environment, you become less tempted by superficial patches and more resolved to support your gut's health.

><

Mara Goes Off on an Unsuspecting
Farmers Market Stand Guy

On Sunday afternoon, Mara stopped by the local Chicago farmers market in La Follette Park. It was the healthiest option possible, or at least it was supposed to be. It was a sunny day, and she passed wooden stands filled with colorful produce and an array of options: honey, citrus, flowers, berries, *oh!*

So much to choose from. All of Dr. Ellis's lectures recommended farmers markets.

The market was, actually, lovely. The sun warmed her skin. Her white dress billowed around her ankles. The scent of sage lofted in the wind. A wild man playing a ukelele sang a throaty tune, and Mara kind of liked it.

She felt chic somehow, gliding between the rustic stands in her lacy sundress. Like she belonged in some all-natural magazine ad. She passed a vegetable stand and admired the forest of lettuce heads and lime-green leaves.

"Are you the farmer?" Mara asked the tall, gangly guy behind the table.

"Nah, I just do this on the side. I'm really a musician," he said with a flourish.

Mara was taken aback. "Oh. Then who grows the produce?"

"This farm is owned by these people . . . Nancy and Ray Stevens. They actually own, like, a few ranches in the state. They're really nice, I heard."

"There's so much lettuce," Mara said. "It must be quite an operation."

"Yeah," the guy shrugged and stuck his hands into his brown corduroy vest pocket. "But there's still, like, all the equipment they use to harvest it, makes it easier. Also there's bug repellent they use. It helps grow more crops."

"Bug repellent?" Mara made a sour expression. "You mean pesticides."

The guy shrugged.

Mara set her jaw. "Pesticides are poison. You know that, right?"

The guy dusted off his wooden table awkwardly, "Yeah, but only a little."

"To the body it's a lot, though," she said louder than she expected. "You know those are endocrine disruptors, right? Those are toxic. They can even cause reproductive harm. I mean, what if I were pregnant?"

The guy stared at her with wide, gray eyes, and slowly tilted his head. "Are you?"

"No, I'm *not!*" she snapped.

The guy made a complicated head gesture.

"Pesticides cause immune system dysfunction, even cancer," Mara said to him. She rubbed a lettuce leaf between her thumb and forefinger. A thin wax coat slid beneath her fingers. It was coated in some invisible pesticide residue or some other toxin. "You know I didn't think I'd have to hunt down organic options at the farmers market, but that's all right. My mood has been better since I started to support my microbiome," she said.

The guy nodded in submissive agreement, as though quietly confirming that she was, in fact, some wild woman.

Mara left and browsed the other stands and picked out half a dozen organic tomatoes, two conventionally grown cucumbers (she could peel them), and a fresh head of lettuce. She imagined her beneficial microbes celebrating.

>————◄

CHAPTER 8

The Gut-Brain Connection

Your gut and your brain have a hidden friendship. Although their bond is not visible, it exists 24/7. Their connection influences how you think, feel, and respond to such things as the box of doughnuts in the office break room. Their relationship explains why stress can send your digestion into a tailspin or why a fast-food PUFS-filled meal can make you cranky and groggy. That is the gut-brain connection. It quietly shapes everything from your mood to your motivation.

It can be easy to think of your brain as being in complete command, sealed off from your gut. However, the gut and brain are in constant dialogue. When your gut has enough Gut Gems, it supplies your body with building blocks to create proper hormonal and neural signals. When toxins or PUFS dominate your diet, they hamper your gut's ability to create Gut Gems and the conversation sours. As a result, you may feel anxious, depressed, or simply not your best.

This chapter will examine the gut-brain relationship. We will look at how stress impacts the microbiome, which influences your mood, and why losing Gut Gems can produce full-body meltdowns.

How a Chatty Gut Can Make or Break Your Day

Do you have a good friend who always checks in to see if you are alright? Yes, you do! One such friend is your gut, which continually communicates with your brain through hormonal signals and neural pathways. When you eat something nourishing, your gut sends a message that says, "Great! This is enough fuel for a busy morning." When you eat an excessive amount of PUFS or skip meals altogether, your gut sends a different notice: "Something is off. We could be in trouble."

This activity happens both chemically (through hormones and messenger molecules) and physically (through the vagus nerve, often described as the highway of gut-brain communication). When all flows smoothly, you have stable energy, stable moods, and fewer cravings. A gut that is nourished appropriately is like a considerate, pleasant roommate who does not disrupt your life. When toxins or stress interfere with your Gut Gems, you instead have a roommate who leaves messes and gets too involved in your personal life. You may be left with poor concentration, twitching nerves, or anxiousness.

The Toxin Trap: How Gut Gem Loss Takes a Toll

Toxins can come from pesticides, plastic food containers, nonstick pans, PUFS, and a steady drip of chronic stress. When they invade your gut environment, those factors chip away at your supply of Gut Gems. In turn, you may have a harder time coping with stress; you may find you experience mental fog or that your mood darkens quickly.

On a positive note, if you feed your body stable saturated fats, your gut can slowly rebuild. Your cells then respond, your gut recovers, and your brain works better.

Stress, Microbiome, and Gut Gems

Stress can be a serious hindrance to health. You might be doing fine, perhaps cooking with butter and coconut oil, and diligently reading labels to avoid PUFS. But if life then tosses a curveball—be it job issues, financial problems, or family drama—your stress levels can soar, and your microbiome feels the tension.

When stress throws your gut microbiome off-balance, it is harder to produce the precious Gut Gems that support your brain's feel-good chemicals. Your gut goes into fight-or-flight mode, which hampers digestion. Gut messengers then tell your brain that things are not okay.

That is why you can experience cravings, anxiety, or both when you are stressed. Can you remember a time when you rummaged through the pantry after a stressful conversation? As you searched for anything to calm your nerves, your gut was in distress, and your brain heard the alarm. Without analyzing why, you did what many people do: You tried to patch the hole with food. Unfortunately, if you turned to processed snacks with PUFS, you created an even greater Gut Gem deficit.

Balancing stress does not demand that you eliminate it altogether. Life doesn't work that way. A better approach is to find ways to keep your gut steady when stress inevitably crops up. Instead of turning to the wrong food, consider releasing tension with mindful breathing, short walks, or moments of silliness.

Keep in mind that if you are under pressure, you especially want to preserve your Gut Gems by eating the right fats. By doing so, you will protect the gut-brain relationship that keeps you levelheaded and capable of handling life's complexities.

How Stress Scrambles Your Gut's Microbial Party

When you are stressed, your body kicks into fight-or-flight mode. The response floods your system with stress hormones such as cortisol. While this is helpful if a wild bear is chasing you, stress hormones are not good for you if they flood your gut on a regular basis.

Chronic stress changes the environment inside your gut in several vital ways:

- **It lowers your gut's barrier defenses**, making it easier for harmful microbes to enter and harder for the good microbes to thrive.
- **It reduces microbial diversity**, meaning you have fewer kinds of helpful bacteria. Imagine your gut ecosystem going from a lush rainforest to a patchy lawn.
- **It favors the growth of less friendly bacteria**, such as certain strains of Clostridium and Escherichia (E. coli). Their presence can lead to more inflammation and digestive troubles.
- **It interferes with gut motility**, slowing things down or speeding them up. Such changes also shift the balance of microbes in the gut.

Stress and Digestion Log

Here is an experiment to help you see just how much stress influences your digestion. Whenever you feel a bit of stress, such as if a traffic jam makes you late for an appointment, pay attention to how your gut feels. Do you get cramps or bloating? Do you feel strangely hungry, craving something crunchy, salty, or sweet? Did you run straight to certain PUFS-filled snacks after a frustrating phone conversation? Did your mood later dip as well? Make note of the kind of stress that triggered you, how you responded, and how your gut reacted.

After a week or two of keeping a record, look back at your notes. You might see unexpected patterns. Once you spot the patterns, you can strategize. Perhaps you schedule a five-minute walk when you sense stress building. The fix can be simple.

Stress and Digestion Log Table

Date and Time	Stress Trigger	Digestion Notes
June 4, 12:30 p.m.	Boss called emergency meeting	Stomach cramps, gas

Fig. 10: Use this space to record the stressors you experience and how your gut reacts to them.

The Vagus Nerve: Your Superhighway

If your gut and brain had a physical phone line, it would be the vagus nerve. This nerve snakes through your body—from the medulla oblongata of the brain stem, down through the neck, chest, and into organs in the abdomen, including the stomach and large intestine—and relays messages in both directions. When your gut is upset, such as from toxins or stress, the vagus nerve picks up the signal and beams it straight to your brain. When your brain interprets the data, the impulse can alter your mood, perhaps by putting you on edge.

On better days, when your gut is content with a good diet, "all is well" signals go through the same vagus nerve. Your brain reads that message and stays in a more relaxed, productive state of mind. You wake up on the "right side of the bed," and everything seems to click into place. Good sleep, balanced hunger cues, and minimal tension can do that. You will feel that way when your vagus nerve is communicating well.

In contrast, when your diet is filled with PUFS or you skip meals because you're too busy, your gut sends a wave of alarm signals. Your brain is suddenly flooded with discomfort and a sense that something is very wrong.

You can encourage a healthy vagus nerve connection through actions as simple as mindful breathing or gentle neck stretches (because the vagus nerve travels through your neck) and avoiding inflammatory foods. All can keep open the nerve's communication lines. If you give your gut the stable fats and daily support it needs, your vagus nerve can deliver mostly good news for a more positive impact on your daily life.

Gut Gems as Brain Boosters

Gut Gems not only preserve the lining of your gut. They also encourage the production of mood-stabilizing and cognition-supporting signals, known as neurotransmitters, that keep your head in a good place.

Neurotransmitters influenced by Gut Gems include:

- **Dopamine:** This is your brain's reward-and-motivation neurotransmitter. It gives you a celebratory feeling when you accomplish something or have fun. Gut Gems can influence dopamine pathways, helping regulate motivation, attention, and movement.

- **GABA (gamma-aminobutyric acid):** Known as the brain's relaxation chemical, GABA calms down nerve activity and helps reduce anxiety, promoting calm and better sleep. Gut Gems increase GABA levels, which can make you feel more grounded and less frazzled.

- **Glutamate:** This powerful excitatory neurotransmitter is your brain's "go" signal. Gut Gems help keep glutamate in check, balancing it with GABA to avoid overstimulation, which could otherwise lead to stress or anxiety.

Gut Gems keep your neurotransmitters healthy. The steady dialogue they maintain with your brain reflects the needs of your daily life.

When your Gut Gems—and thus your neurotransmitters—are running low, you will experience a difference. Brain fog, low-grade anxiety, and sugar cravings, for instance, can all be signs that your gut is struggling to produce enough Gut Gems to stay on track.

A Damaged Gut Harms Your Brain

Of all the important ideas to take with you, remember that your gut-brain axis is the core of how your body manages stress, processes daily experiences, and keeps your head in a good place. When your gut is in disrepair, your brain pays the price—and vice versa. Your body will function better on every level once you protect your gut-brain axis through managing stress and making the right food choices.

Over time, you'll see a new mental baseline emerge, one where your mind feels sharper, your moods more balanced, and your overall sense of "I can handle this" grows. A big part of this process is forgiveness—of yourself, your body, your slipups. The gut isn't a machine; it's more like a garden. Sometimes you forget to water it, or you get a nasty round of weeds. If you approach your task of cleaning up the mess and nurturing the rest with patience, feeding it consistently with stable fats and better emotional habits, it can bounce back gracefully.

———

Mara Hates Aunt Linda's Casserole and Doesn't Know How to Tell Her

Mara arrived at Aunt Linda's house in the Bronzeville neighborhood of Chicago, where her family cookout was in full swing. Mara stood at the edge of the lawn, tentative. She peered around the corner of her aunt's house toward the tables full of desserts, hot dogs, potato salad, barbecue sauce, and cheesecake. She took a deep breath and walked past the lawn chairs over to the food table with a bowl of roasted veggies. The chatter of lively conversation among her family floated across the backyard with a warm breeze.

Aunt Linda's signature dish sat in a giant pan in the middle of all the other dishes: a savory potato casserole. It smelled of cheese dipped in fried bread and drenched in canola oil, because that's what it was. This casserole was the stuff of family legend. Everyone praised it so much, it became known as The Casserole, as if all other casseroles were unworthy of the name.

Aunt Linda took her place by the food table, wearing a blue gingham dress and looking as though she had stepped out of a '70s cookbook.

Mara's family took turns piling Aunt Linda's casserole onto their plates. Aunt Linda stood by and smiled approvingly.

Little Jimmy took a scoop; Aunt Linda patted his head.

Auntie May took a scoop; Aunt Linda bowed a little, nodding.

Grandma Tati took a scoop, and Aunt Linda gushed. She did that thing when someone laughs with their mouth closed and smiles at the same time.

Mara stepped up to the dinner table and placed some of her own roasted vegetables on her plate. Really, with her new diet, she could not eat anything else.

"Forgetting something?" Aunt Linda cooed.

"Hmmm?" Mara turned to her.

"Your casserole," Aunt Linda blushed. "It's your favorite. Or as you said when you were six, 'My fave-ie.'"

Mara's face froze into a half smile. "When I was six, right," Mara awkwardly patted around the table, hoping Aunt Linda would turn away or something.

She didn't.

"Go on," Aunt Linda pressed, with a firm smile.

"What?" Mara said stupidly.

In a brief, insane moment, frustration flashed over Aunt Linda's face. She looked horrible, something of a monster. But then the flash was gone and her expression snapped back into a smile. "Oh, don't worry, pumpkin. I'll help you."

Aunt Linda scooped the biggest, heaviest serving of casserole Mara had ever seen onto Mara's plate, right on top of her roasted vegetables.

"Thank you," Mara said artificially and walked away with stiff steps.

Mara sat at a picnic table beside her nephew Thomas and a crying baby and stared at the casserole. In years past, it would have been delicious, but now it didn't even look that appealing. Besides, the bloat and mental fog that would follow would make her regret the decision tomorrow.

"You're not gonna eat it?" Little Thomas asked discreetly, chewing.

Mara glanced down at him and shook her head.

"Good thing you didn't tell Aunt Linda," he smacked his lips.

"Yeah," she cracked a smile down at him. "You know what, since starting my new diet, I don't feel as angry anymore. I'm not as stressed in situations like these."

"That's good," Little Thomas said, chewing casserole, "Cuz you get angry a lot."

✦

CHAPTER 9

Your Gut's Built-In Intelligence for Weight Loss

Weight-loss advice can be downright confusing. Some blame calories or carbs, others blame saturated fats such as butter. The truth is that PUFS are not your friend, whether you want to lose weight or not. Your gut craves real nourishment and a balanced environment to naturally regulate hunger, fat storage, and weight. To understand how your gut bacteria and the Gut Gems they produce can help you lose weight, we will look deep within your colon, where L cells work their magic.

Your L cells are tucked within your gut lining. When they detect nutrients, they jump into action, releasing hormones that help regulate your appetite and keep your digestion running smoothly. You can think of your L cells as the calm and collected servers in a busy restaurant kitchen. Unfazed by all the activity and demands, they efficiently keep the orders flowing.

When your diet is poor, your L cells become overwhelmed and communication lines go fuzzy. That is how hunger cues spin out of control and snack cravings move in. The Gut Gem butyrate is a key player in this system. It teams up with L cells, so your gut and your hormones work in tandem. Their synergy matters because your appetite determines the environment of your gut. Support your L cells and you are telling your whole system to rest, digest, and run a tight ship. Neglect them or bombard them with PUFS-filled junk foods and you end up with frayed signaling, wild cravings, and a gut that cannot function optimally.

Balancing Hormones Without the Hype

Two of the most influential hormones created in your gut that dictate hunger and metabolism are peptide YY and glucagon-like peptide-1—known more simply as PYY and GLP-1.

PYY is the hormone that signals fullness and satisfaction after a meal, while GLP-1 helps manage blood sugar levels and encourages your stomach to empty at a reasonable pace. When the two hormones are in balance, you stay satisfied longer and experience fewer energy crashes.

Put simply, these two hormones are watchful monitors over your metabolic system.

The big twist is a pharmaceutical approach that mimics GLP-1. The brand Ozempic is one of several such drugs out there. Unfortunately, the synthetic drug comes with a long list of side effects. Topping the list is the drug's ability to mask problems related to your overall gut health. Rather than paying top dollar to trick your system artificially, you can get similar benefits by supporting your natural L cells to churn out the hormones you need in the right amounts.

How do you do that? You feed and nurture your gut environment by focusing on butyrate as well as by dropping the processed foods that are messing up your internal ecosystem. Once you help your L cells thrive, your own PYY and GLP-1 levels can self-balance. You will not have to rely on outside synthetic solutions. You already have everything you need built right into your system, if you help your gut do its job.

You already met the *Akkermansia* protein Amuc_1100 back in chapter 3, where we explained how this protein helps zip up the tight junctions between your intestinal cells. Another protein carried by this bacterium is called P9. It's a messenger protein that whispers directly to your gut's L-cells—the hormone factories that control appetite, blood sugar, and energy use. When P9 shows up, L-cells pump out GLP-1 naturally. And, unlike GLP-1 weight loss drugs, P9 doesn't hijack anything. It works within your own system, coaxing your body to make just enough GLP-1 at the right time. No gas pedal jammed to the floor. No brute force. Just a nudge in the language your body already understands.

Healing from Within: Butyrate's Core Mechanisms

The link between butyrate and your colon resembles a great romance. They are better together. Butyrate, made by friendly gut microbes, is quickly consumed as fuel by your colonocytes—the cells that line the inner walls of your colon and play a key role in keeping your gut healthy.

Think of connecting your phone to a superfast and reliable charger; the battery is replenished quickly and fully. Similarly, the energy source provided by butyrate keeps the colon well fueled and running at top speed. It also maintains the gut lining and helps your L cells do their job effectively.

When your gut bacteria break down food remnants, they release the butyrate that your colonocytes rely on for their daily energy. Picture your colonocytes as little workers in a well-lit workshop; see them hammering away at tasks such as hormone signaling, forming a barrier between your gut and the outside world, and managing synergy with your immune system. Give your colonocytes enough butyrate, and they bloom into unstoppable gatekeepers that support your entire body.

If your diet is brimming with PUFS, your gut flora is imbalanced with an overabundance of the wrong microbes. The result will be less butyrate, fewer Gut Gems, and a slump in colonocyte productivity.

Fortunately, tipping the balance back in your favor is within your reach. Your task is to phase out PUFS, replace them with stable, saturated fats, and keep an eye on boosting your butyrate production. Just remember: Stable fats complement—rather than replace—fiber in butyrate production. Without fermentable fibers, your microbes can't make enough butyrate, no matter how stable your fat sources are. Over time, your colonocytes perk up, your L cells start celebrating, and your entire GI tract can breathe a sigh of relief.

Each step leads to a natural cascade of improvements, including less bloating, more predictable bowel movements, and better control of your cravings. If weight loss is a goal, you will benefit from not eating on impulse. After all, when your gut and brain are on speaking terms, your body can more easily figure out how much is enough.

Your Body's Built-In Healing Loops

Butyrate and your weight exist within a beautiful circle: A robust supply of butyrate helps tighten your gut barrier, which lowers inflammation. Less inflammation, in turn, frees your L cells to produce more appetite-balancing hormones. The cyclical pattern fosters health from the inside out. Your system does not need to rely on external fixes.

When your colonocytes function well, your immune cells are not on red alert over every little trigger. The calm environment makes it easier for PYY and GLP-1 to do their jobs, helping you maintain a comfortable sense of fullness after meals. If you were to slip up and indulge in something questionable, your well-toned system could handle it without a meltdown.

How Your Gut Regulates Appetite: The L Cell and Butyrate Connection

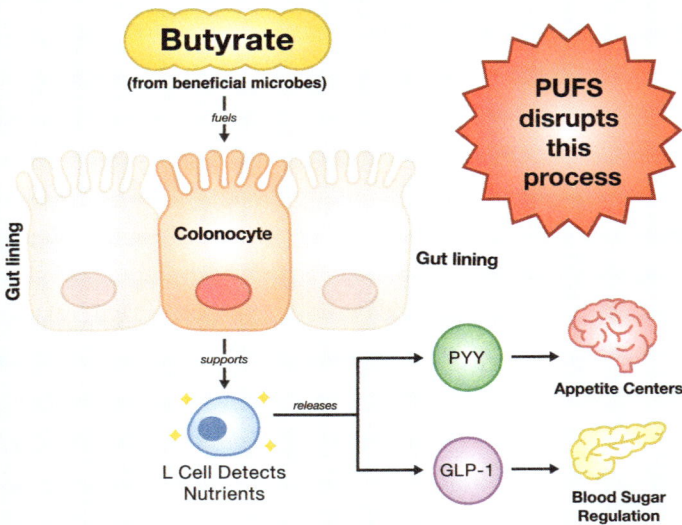

Fig. 11: Butyrate kicks off a cycle that helps regulate both appetite and blood sugar, boosting metabolic health.

An irritated gut equates to an irritated immune system, which can lead to full-body distress. Simply put, an inflamed gut cannot effectively absorb nutrients or regulate hunger. Butyrate is essentially your gut's personal meditation coach, gently reminding your gut's immune cells to keep calm. Your hormones then work better, and you reduce random aches, cravings, and midafternoon slumps. Also, a calm, balanced environment ties right back into your L cells' capacity to release messages that you are full and satisfied after meals.

Why Restrictive Diets Rarely Work

If you have ever tried extreme diets, especially ones that count every macronutrient down to the last gram, you know the frustration. Sure, you may have found that you could muscle your way through such regimens for a month or two, but life eventually happened. Some event—maybe a friend's birthday party or a family vacation—reduced your willpower to a single crumb of cake. You reverted to old habits because you never addressed the root cause of your cravings: an imbalanced gut environment.

When you nurture your L cells and support butyrate production, you effectively tell your body that you trust in its built-in design to regulate your appetite. This is a far cry from ignoring hunger pangs and forcing no-fat lunches. Instead, you embrace stable fats such as butter or coconut oil while kicking PUFS out the door. As you learn to trust your body's signals, your appetite will feel more predictable and less adversarial.

This approach also liberates you from guilt cycles. You are probably familiar with giving in to an unhealthy craving and then beating yourself up and vowing to be more disciplined the next day. That mental ping-pong is exhausting.

Instead, you can experience a peaceful relationship with food when your improved gut environment gradually recalibrates your sense of portion sizes. You can feel satiated from eating real foods and crave less processed junk. The self-sustaining loop of feeling good and enjoying food freely certainly beats a restriction-based mentality.

A Closer Look at Habitual Eating Patterns

Ever wonder why you sometimes raid the fridge at odd hours, nibbling on stuff you don't particularly love? It could be a sign of hormones gone haywire. If your gut and brain are out of sync, your body interprets stress or emotional dips as a call for food. By reinforcing your L cells with a diet that fosters butyrate production, you break that cycle.

The imbalance does not always show up as hunger. Sometimes it manifests as strange anxiety or irritability that eases only after you snack on something with a lot of refined sugar, particularly fructose. You may have felt "hangry" and craved quick-burning carbs. Odd cravings are your body's way of signaling that your deeper regulation systems are not functioning optimally. Once you restore those systems, food no longer has to be an emotional crutch.

You may notice other benefits as well, such as clearer thinking, improved skin, and better mood regulation. The positives are all connected to the chain reaction that starts with butyrate and other Gut Gems. When your colonocytes and L cells have the right environment, you benefit from the inside-out.

Boost Your Gut's Potential

The plan to revive your gut is surprisingly straightforward:

1. Reduce or eliminate PUFS.

2. Embrace stable, nourishing fats such as butter, ghee, tallow, and/or coconut oil as PUFS alternatives.

3. Consider an enteric-coated *postbiotic Akkermansia* supplement to accelerate epithelial repair and tight-junction support.

4. Consider increasing your intake of C15:0 to accelerate PUFS removal and detox, as discussed in my book *Fat Cure*.

5. Consider adding an *Akkermansia* probiotic.

If a Drug Is Popular, Does that Mean It's Safe?

Before we move on, let's circle back to GLP-1 drugs for a moment. Imagine you are sitting in your favorite coffee shop, scrolling through social media. Eventually you find a post about a so-called miracle drug that melts pounds away. Of course, you must be willing to stomach the side effects and fork over some serious cash. Like so many who stumble across the ad, you are curious, especially if you have struggled with weight and energy for years. Mainstream marketing will pitch you a thousand reasons to hop aboard the Ozempic spaceship. Before you do, step back and consider the broader picture. Make sure you understand what your gut needs. Most importantly, take a good look at how today's popular drugs have seized the spotlight.

Ozempic and other GLP-1 agonists are lauded by celebrities, influencers, and many others who would like to drop extra weight without complicated diets. The drug's rise to stardom is staggering. We hear about it on podcasts and news segments. We see ads in popular magazines. According to reports, one in four people with type 2 diabetes have tried GLP-1 agonists such as Ozempic. Even more startling is a 700 percent surge in usage among those *without* a diagnosis of diabetes.

That star power, though, casts some big shadows: lumps at the injection site, risk to your vision, and a wallet screaming for mercy. And for what? A short-term solution that often leaves you worse off than when you started. When something skyrockets that fast, the product is either a genuine breakthrough, a result of hyped marketing, or both.

At first glance, the quick fix is appealing. Rather than reworking your daily habits, you can keep your drive-through breakfasts and PUFS-filled snacks and hope the shots prevent the usual consequences. A way to cheat the system certainly seems easier than balancing hormones, appetite, and your gut. But you might wind up paying for the convenience in unexpected ways. Yes, a medication such as Ozempic can help lower blood sugar and shave off pounds, but at what cost? If you want some legitimate reasons to be concerned, pay attention to the itemized list of disclaimers in drug commercials.

The Risks and Costs of GLP-1 Weight-Loss Drugs

The financial commitment is another issue for most people. The medications are pricey, and insurance coverage is often lacking. If you could no longer afford the drug, would you also lose your progress overnight?

The possibility of developing a dependence on weight-loss drugs is another real problem. Many people rely on medications for vital reasons, but is taking a costly drug such as Ozempic to drop clothing sizes justified? The answer is personal, but the better strategy for most individuals and their bank accounts is to eat the stable fats and nourishment their bodies require to produce their own hormone-balancing magic.

Remember, in the right environment, the gut naturally creates the same appetite-regulating signals that GLP-1 and PYY produce. GLP-1 is essentially an internal accountant that keeps track of how much you have eaten and tells your brain to dial down hunger if you are full. It also teams up with insulin, ensuring your energy is not dropping due to a sugar imbalance within an hour of eating a meal. PYY helps you skip impulse eating when you should be satisfied. The two hormones work together, naturally, without risk of undesirable side effects.

People often discover that once they leave medication behind, old habits roar back with a vengeance. Then they feel more lost than before. To avoid the ups and downs, stay away from short-term, synthetic hacks and gravitate to nurturing a system that fosters natural, physical, and emotional harmony.

Natural Gut Hormone Regulation vs. GLP-1 Agonist Drugs

	Natural GLP-1 PYY Regulation	GLP-1 Agonist Drugs (e.g., Ozempic)
Source	Healthy gut/L Cells fueled by butyrate	Synthetic injection
Mechanism	Natural signaling through the gut's own hormone production	Mimics hormone action artificially
Side Effects	Minimal or none	Lumps, vision issues, gastrointestinal distress, etc.
Cost	Requires lifestyle and dietary changes	High financial cost
Sustainability	High—can be maintained through consistent healthy habits	Dependent on ongoing use, access, and affordability

Fig. 12: A side-by-side comparison of the features of managing your GLP-1 levels naturally versus using a GLP-1 agonist drug

The emotional break from putting all your faith in quick fixes can be liberating. What a relief not to be stuck on endless medication! In a world that rewards instant gratification, a little patience goes a long way. If you have sworn off medication-based shortcuts, the best way to maintain your momentum is through consistency with stable fats.

Seeing Your Body as a Collaborative Partner

Of course, we are all human. Sometimes we stress, which can lead to mindlessly chomping on a great temptation. Whether it is peanut butter and crackers or a bag of chocolate-dipped toffee, slipups happen. That is life! The key is not to let a single "off" day snowball into a total meltdown.

Self-correction is a lifesaver. In time, you will feel the difference between feeding yourself butyrate-building choices and bogging it down with PUFS. You will not only recognize how quickly your body bounces back from occasional indulgences, but you will also avoid many regretful moments after "falling off the wagon." The critical shift to self-correction indicates you are listening to your gut's feedback. If you sense you are bloated or extra sluggish after a "cheat" meal, you will know what triggered it and change course.

─────

Mara Takes a Hike and Says No to the Latest Weight-Loss Drug

Dawn lit the morning sky in pink and blue, and Mara laced up her boots for an early hike in the nearby hills just outside of Chicago. With each step, stones crunched beneath her boots. Fresh air mixed with the scents of pine and dusty earth filled her lungs. Her mind felt sharper, her body invigorated.

Mara paused at the peak—mountains and rolling green hills expanded in every direction. *What a beautiful world,* she thought. She leaned on the trail post and scuffed the dirt with her boot. Her feet didn't even ache. *My body is stronger than ever.*

Mara reached into her pocket and found the GLP-1 receptor agonist pill Sarah had given her. At the gym, Sarah had urged her to try it and said it would give her that edge she'd been looking for. But Mara felt conflicted about it. According to Dr. Ellis, her body could make the same chemical markers naturally.

She toyed with it in her hand. It was white, simple, and seemed so small, so harmless. It would be easy to swallow. She could do it right now.

Mara brought the pill to her lips and recalled Dr. Ellis's lecture about how these pills could have side effects. Bad side effects. Mara blushed and stuffed it away all at once: "What am I thinking? It could ruin my progress."

Mara shook her head and started back down the trail, thinking, *I've come too far in letting my body heal. I trust it. For now, real foods and supplements are best. I won't sabotage my progress.*

———

CHAPTER 10

Gut Gems and Neurological Health

Have you heard that a damaged gut could play a role in brain disorders and diseases? The idea is new to many. For years, the link was not directly addressed. Instead, the medical community focused on quick-fix medications that target symptoms without giving thought to gut health.

Nevertheless, a growing body of insightful research shows that low levels of Gut Gems often coincide with conditions such as Alzheimer's and Parkinson's diseases. In some cases, the presence of amyloid plaques or motor issues appear to be directly tied to a poor gut environment. For too long, science has focused solely on the brain without considering the gut's role in shaping many of the body's neural signals.

In a perfect world, your beneficial microbes generate enough butyrate to keep your cells loaded with Gut Gems. Under current conditions, day after day, they are more likely hammered by PUFS-filled products and/or toxins. Over time, a decreased production of Gut Gems leaves your colonocytes too drained to keep everything balanced.

Meanwhile, your brain may begin to wave red flags. Warning signs include brain fog, memory lapses, or moments of confusion. If you're like most people, you probably chalk up such issues to aging, but failing memory, even in your senior years, is far from inevitable. Of course, a single spoonful of butyrate will not reverse neurological disorders overnight. But if you suspect your daily diet could be fueling your cognitive challenges, whether an early sign of memory loss or a deeper degenerative shift, let it be a wake-up call to move away from quick-fix solutions and toward a gut-first mindset.

Most importantly, your beneficial gut bacteria must make enough Gut Gems. If they don't, your brain cells will not have what they need for proper function, no matter how many alternative therapies you try.

Butyrate's Neuroprotective Edge

Unexplainable fatigue and random aches are both possible signs that inflammation is stuck in high gear. And chronic inflammation does not stop at your joints or digestive tract. It can also slip past your gut's boundaries and stir up trouble in your brain cells. Like a steady hand that keeps your immune signals under control, butyrate can calm the same inflammatory pathways in your body that are frazzled in your brain.

Some research points to butyrate's ability to dismantle the protein clumps, known as beta-amyloid plaques, which build up in degenerative conditions. This finding is a vital breakthrough if you are concerned about age-related cognitive decline. A healthy supply of Gut Gems can help your body keep protein buildup in check. You may have watched friends or family chase medication after medication, each tackling a narrow slice of the problem without restoring the gut environment the brain needs. So many people also bounce from doctor to doctor, searching for the next big fix. If they were short on Gut Gems from the start, all those external aids could not replicate what a well-fueled gut does naturally.

Of course, no single factor dictates the onset of complex conditions. But ignoring your gut's role is like going into a marathon with only one shoe. Why not give yourself every advantage to come out ahead?

Butyrate is not necessarily a cure-all, but if you are concerned about cognitive decline, ignoring your gut's supply of Gut Gems might be the biggest oversight. Over time, ensuring your colonocytes have enough stable fats and minimal PUFS can reduce the load that accelerates plaque formation or intensifies motor symptoms. Imagine gaining more freedom to enjoy life with less time worrying about losing mental ground too soon!

How Butyrate Protects Against Neuroinflammation

Low levels of Gut Gems can turn up the volume on neuroinflammation, which is widely recognized as a key factor in the development and progression of a wide range of neurodegenerative diseases, including Alzheimer's disease, Parkinson's disease, and multiple sclerosis. Therefore, if you do not produce enough Gut Gems, the likelihood of developing neurodegenerative diseases increases. Also, if you already have one of the diseases, the symptoms may worsen.

Like a calm-down coach for your body's inflammation team, butyrate helps maintain peace by blocking a key pathway called NF-κB (nuclear factor kappa-light-chain-enhancer of activated B cells). For a visual, imagine the pathway as a drill sergeant that rallies the body to produce a variety of inflammatory substances. When butyrate comes in and mitigates NF-κB, it helps stop the body from making too many inflammatory molecules (called cytokines), which in turn promote neuroinflammation and interfere with brain function.

Another way butyrate supports brain health is by taking on enzymes called HDACs (histone deacetylases), which decide how your genes are expressed. Think of HDACs as referees who determine how players in a youth league will engage. Will they allow the kids to aggressively tackle one another, or will the referees keep opposing players in check? By calming down your HDAC referees, butyrate helps your brain cells switch on the good genes that reduce inflammation. They also turn down the ones that stir it up.

Interestingly, in a study with animals that had Alzheimer's-like symptoms, butyrate helped reduce beta-amyloid plaques by up to 40 percent. As a result, the animals experienced better memory and thinking ability.

Emotional Well-Being and Mood

You have likely experienced days when your mood dropped for no clear reason. Perhaps you chalked it up to stress or lack of sleep. If you are living on processed foods filled with PUFS, your colonocytes are essentially being starved of butyrate. The lack can inhibit the brain's ability to regulate mood chemicals such as dopamine, which can lead to or worsen anxiety and depression.

In short, supporting your gut health provides emotional stability. Stress resilience also often improves. Additionally, those 3:00 p.m. energy slumps should be minimal or nonexistent.

Ignoring gut health often creates a cycle of quick fixes that treat symptoms. External solutions such as pills, however, cannot support your body forever. Eventually, if your gut remains neglected, your mood will probably not remain stable. On the bright side, by supporting your gut's ability to produce butyrate and other Gut Gems, you may find your mental clarity and emotional stability return naturally. If you were taking a prescription, you may no longer need it.

Brain-Boosting Snack Ideas

You may love the idea of a stable gut and a calm mind but cringe at the thought of complicated meal plans. Rest assured, it can be as simple as scrambling your morning eggs in butter or adding a splash of cream (or a dollop of coconut oil or unsalted butter) to your coffee or tea. Just remember to skip fiber-dense foods if your gut is in a fragile state. Instead, lean on butyrate-rich or butyrate-boosting options, like full-fat dairy and simple homemade recipes with stable fats.

Foods that Contain Butyrate Directly

The following foods naturally have a small amount of butyrate:
- **Butter,** especially from grass-fed cows, is the richest direct source of butyrate.
- **Ghee,** or clarified butter, is high in butyrate and easier to digest than butter.
- **Parmesan cheese** and other aged cheeses have a bit of butyrate, too.
- **Full-fat dairy products,** such as whole milk, cream, and yogurt (especially if fermented), are good sources.

Foods that Help Your Gut Make Butyrate

The following foods are rich in prebiotic fibers that feed butyrate-producing bacteria:

- **Oats**, often enjoyed as a cozy bowl of oatmeal, are great fuel for your gut.
- **Bananas**, especially slightly green ones, have resistant starch.
- **Apples** are full of pectin, a fiber your gut loves.
- **Sweet potatoes** are rich in fiber. Their antioxidants and vitamins also reduce inflammation and strengthen the gut lining.
- **Garlic** and **onions** help balance gut bacteria.

Snack Ideas to Boost Butyrate Naturally

- A small bowl of Greek yogurt with banana slices and oats
- Whole grain toast with grass-fed butter or ghee
- Apple slices with nut butter (look for brands without added oils)
- Roasted chickpeas or sweet potato fries
- A Parmesan crisp (or two) for a cheesy, crunchy treat
- Overnight oats with berries

Gut Game—Cognitive Longevity Challenge

If you like the idea of turning your diet adjustments into a game, consider the Cognitive Longevity Challenge. Each day, see how many times you can fit in butyrate-friendly staples. Maybe you add some Parmesan cheese to your usual veggie omelet for breakfast and make a ghee-based sauce for the fish you prepare for dinner. Each successful swap earns you a point. Keep track. At the end of the week, reward yourself with something that is not food. Take a relaxing bath, for instance, or plan an evening with friends. Also, track your mental clarity and mood. Jot down if you felt more relaxed at work or if you powered through the afternoon with enough energy.

At the end of your challenge, reflect on whether you noticed tangible benefits. Did you have better memory and a happier mood? No injection or pill can reward you so well!

Food and Mood Log

Date and Time	Food	Mood Notes
June 10 7:30 a.m.	Coffee with a little coconut oil and egg scrambled in butter	Focused, calm

Fig. 13: Use this log to track how what you eat affects how you feel mentally and emotionally.

Key Takeaway—Protect Your Brain by Healing Your Gut

You might be tempted to pick up the latest memory supplement or a pricey medication if you sense your brain is not as sharp as it once was. But remember, if your gut is starved of butyrate, you are already on shaky ground. Overloading your system with PUFS or ignoring toxins will starve your colonocytes of the Gut Gems that keep your neural circuits running smoothly.

Instead, consider fueling them from the inside out. Once your gut thrives, your brain usually follows suit. Mind-body synergy beats any medication's claims of magical results. So, remember, each time you feed your gut, you feed your mind.

━━

Mara Keeps Her Cool at the Zoo and Gets Promoted

Mara drove to work in her black SUV one morning, on her way to the Chicago Zoo offices. Mara spoke on the phone with her mother, who was worried about Aunt Linda.

"She's acting ridiculous!" her mother's voice resounded through the car speaker. Her mother described how Aunt Linda had displayed some memory lapses lately. Apparently she cooked several casseroles and forgot she had made them. She kept handing them out to her neighbors over and over. It was the beginning of cognitive decline. Mara could just imagine all the bottled dressings, canned fried onions, and other seed-oil-heavy ingredients her aunt used in her recipes. *Of course,* Mara thought, *there might be a connection.*

"You know ever since I've started my new diet avoiding seed oils, I haven't had as much brain fog," Mara said, and explained how the gut-brain connection was more interconnected than she had realized.

Mara hung up, pulled into work, and chewed her piece of toast slathered in butter to boost her gut's access to butyrate's "magic." She savored the creamy taste.

At work in the Chicago Zoo offices, Mara calmly organized her desk without the usual hurried scramble. Her work phone rang constantly, but instead of an adrenaline rush, she felt a steady hum of energy.

Mara was even forced by her boss to give a last-minute presentation on the new orangutan exhibit for the city council members. Instead of panicking, her mood stayed steady. She felt confident. Instead of reaching for a snack to calm her nerves, she sipped tea and nibbled on cheese. To her amazement, she gave her presentation quite easily. She spoke confidently and clicked through the presentation slides easily in the long meeting room, showing the various new animals. Her voice was calm. She was grounded, and she was herself.

Right after the meeting, once all the city council members left, the zoo director stopped her with a hand on her way out.

"Mara, wait," he spluttered.

She turned.

"That was fantastic," he stroked his white mustache. "I'm really sorry to have dropped that on you last-minute. Didn't mean to. But you've been working so hard. You know these exhibits inside out."

"Thanks," Mara softened.

"We're going to give you a raise," he muttered casually. "And a promotion. You're worth it. You earned it."

><

CHAPTER 11

Gut Gems Affect
Every Part of Your Body

It is easy to chalk up frequent colds, energy dips, and other illnesses to "getting older" or "having too much stress" without suspecting the underlying reason: a lack of Gut Gems, which influence every aspect of your health. Most people try to fix one symptom at a time, maybe by taking an over-the-counter allergy medication for their constant sniffles, chasing a new miracle pill to help lower their blood sugar, and relying on caffeine to give them an energy boost when fatigue strikes. All the while, each ill likely has the same root—a battered gut lacking in Gut Gems. Failing to address the underlying cause is like bailing water out of a boat while ignoring the hole in the hull.

If your gut cells are starved of what they need, don't give up. You can step in and restore your gut environment by kicking out PUFS, adding stable fats, and eating more foods that allow your colonocytes to produce more Gut Gems. Once that happens, your body can tap into the synergy that becomes available to lift everything from your immune function to your daily energy.

How Immunity Thrives on Gut Gems

When you think of immunity, you might picture white blood cells zapping invaders. That happens, but your gut plays a large part. One of the real heroes in your gut are the regulatory T cells (Tregs), which help your system decide when to fight off actual threats. They also determine when to calm down. The regulatory function of Tregs keeps your body from being continuously inflamed. Interestingly, Tregs flourish on Gut Gems.

Your colonocytes, when given butyrate, are more likely to produce enough Gut Gems to support Tregs. If you starve your colonocytes by overconsuming PUFS or toxins, you sabotage these immune modulators. That can leave your system more prone to overreact and possibly set you up for seasonal allergies. It can also underreact and leave you wide open to every germ that crosses your path. Over time, problems can migrate from chronic sniffles to inflammatory issues, going from bad to worse.

Restoring your Gut Gem output can give your Tregs a stable environment, making your immune response more measured and less prone to extremes. Your immunity then achieves balance.

The benefits of immunity reach organs throughout the body, including the brain, heart, and lungs. Without inflammation in the brain, cognitive function improves. In the heart, Gut Gems help keep blood vessels healthy and flexible, which supports good blood pressure and reduces the risk of heart disease. In the lungs, Gut Gems lower inflammation, which may help with breathing issues such as asthma or chronic lung conditions.

How Gut Gems Shape Your Metabolism

When you eat something sweet, the ideal response is for your pancreas to release insulin, which then shuttles blood sugar out of circulation and into your cells to counter the effect. Consequently your blood sugar does not spike. However, if your gut is low on Gut Gems, your insulin sensitivity can drop, and your body will have a harder time clearing out extra glucose. As a result, your insulin levels will remain high. This is known as insulin resistance.

Insulin resistance affects your daily energy, how you store body fat, and how you bounce back from surges of sugar intake. If your gut is starved of Gut Gems, the synergy that should help your cells respond to insulin can break down. You may, in turn, notice an increase in stored body fat and energy dips after mealtimes.

When your insulin function is steady, you are less likely to store fat in all the wrong places and more inclined to maintain constant energy throughout the day. Also, your body can handle refined fructose and other nutrients with greater ease.

In contrast, quick-fix approaches, such as appetite-suppression medications, only hush your desire to eat. They ignore how your system manages food once you are digesting it. If your gut still produces some Gut Gems, you may maintain or lose weight over the short term, but you can imagine what happens when you stop taking the prescription. Instead of going down that dead-end route, adding butyrate to produce Gut Gems can give your entire metabolic system a tune-up.

Body-Wide Effects of Gut Gems

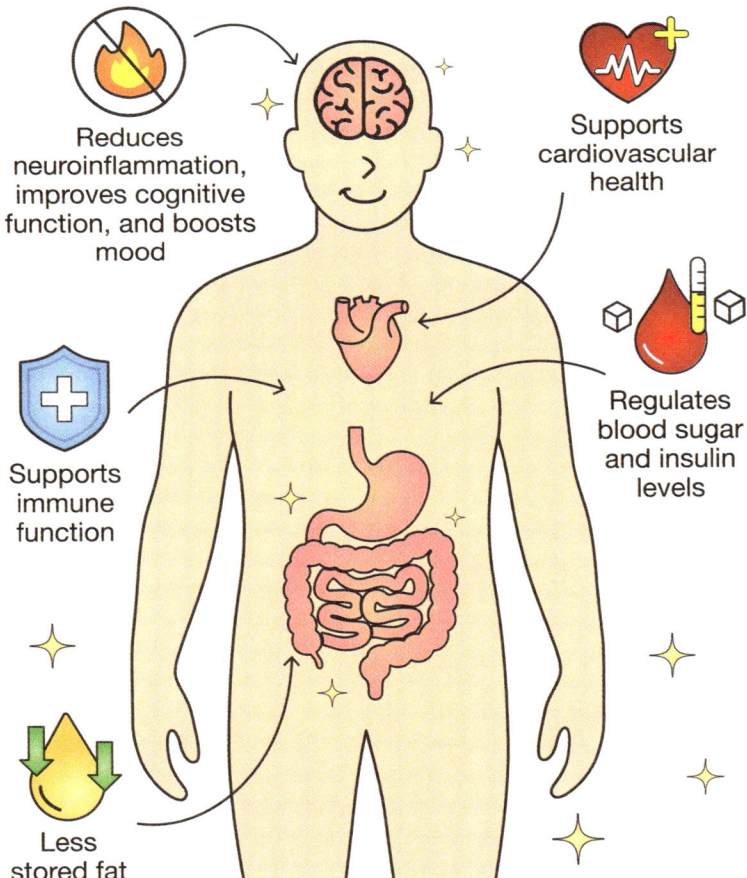

Reduces neuroinflammation, improves cognitive function, and boosts mood

Supports cardiovascular health

Supports immune function

Regulates blood sugar and insulin levels

Less stored fat

Fig. 14: Gut Gems travel throughout the body, positively influencing your health in multiple ways.

Systemic Health Quiz

To see if your overall system is feeling the effects of a gut low on Gut Gems, answer the following questions:

- Do you often experience allergy symptoms (stuffy nose, watery eyes, itchy skin, or fatigue)?

- Do you notice that certain foods leave you bloated, gassy, or crampy—or that some personal care products trigger redness, itching, or rashes?

- Do you catch more viruses (cold, sniffles, flu, or stomach bugs) than you believe is normal?

- Has your weight increased despite your best efforts?

- Do you experience regular sugar cravings?

- Does your energy regularly drop for no apparent reason?

- Would your friends or loved ones describe you as moody?

Every "yes" or "not sure" answer could be a sign that your gut environment needs a little help. It does not mean you are doomed or that you must throw out everything in your fridge. You should, however, keep an eye on your daily choices. Are you leaning on stable fats or allowing PUFS to slip in at every meal? Are you still microwaving convenience items that are full of additives? If so, your colonocytes probably need some relief.

PUFS-Free Convenience Swaps for Busy Days

These fast, simple, PUFS-free options can help you sidestep seed oils—even on your busiest days:

- **Hard-boiled eggs:** Quick to prepare in batches and packed with protein. One caveat: Factory-farmed eggs can contain relatively high amounts of LA, thanks to the chickens being fed high-PUFS diets. For minimal PUFS, seek out eggs from organically raised hens that have been fed an intentionally low-PUFS diet.

- **Full-fat plain Greek yogurt:** Creamy, filling, and free from added oils.

- **Fresh fruit (apples, bananas, grapes, berries, oranges):** Portable, prep-free, and naturally PUFS-free.

- **Raw or steamed veggies (carrots, celery, cucumbers, bell peppers):** Pair with oil-free hummus or eat plain for a crunchy, satisfying snack.

- **Air-fried baked potato (plain or topped with butter or salsa):** Quick and filling; top with a pat of butter for C15:0.

- **Stovetop popcorn:** A simple snack you can make in minutes. Add melted butter, herbs, or sea salt for flavor.

- **Full-fat cottage cheese with side of fruit or fresh berries:** High-protein; great as a dip or quick bite.

- **Frozen banana bites**: Slice a ripe banana and dip the slices in full-fat yogurt, then freeze until firm for a PUFS-free treat. For a richer, sweeter twist, dip the banana slices in dark chocolate (70–85 percent cacao), melted with a little coconut oil, then freeze. While dark chocolate does contain a small amount of PUFS—about 0.3 to 0.4 gram per 1-ounce serving, mostly from LA—it's a minimal trade-off for an occasional antioxidant-rich indulgence.

———

Sarah Comes Over for Dinner and Notices Mara's New Mood

At home, Mara stirred ghee into her vegetable-sauté dinner and Sarah sat with the cat on the white sofa, watching. Mara flipped a switch on the radio and turned up Mariah Carey's Christmas song. "I love this one!" Mara laughed and danced with the wooden spoon in her hand. "It doesn't have to be Christmas to listen to this song."

Sarah could hardly believe her eyes as Mara danced in her kitchen. "Okay, I have never seen you with this much energy before."

"Try it," Mara twirled, and forked a piece of chicken for Sarah. "I even got a promotion at work."

"Really?" Sarah beamed and tried the chicken. "It sure beats my nasty protein shake. I always hated those canned shakes but never wanted to complain."

"Why not?" Mara stirred the veggies in her saucepan. "It's gross! Complain about it!"

Sarah cradled the cat sweetly and nodded at Mara. "It's like you're an entirely new person. In a good way, though."

Mara filled their plates with veggies, and they chatted about their new gym outfits and debated whether it was better to deadlift barefoot or in shoes. Most importantly, they talked about Mara's new energy.

"Whatever you're doing," Sarah said, "I want to do it, too."

———

CHAPTER 12

Diet and Gut Health

For decades, health gurus pushed the idea that fiber is the answer to all digestive problems. Granted, fiber can address many issues, but only if the gut microbiome is balanced and healthy. As mentioned, if your gut is actively sabotaged with toxins and PUFS, your beneficial microbes can easily become outnumbered by bad ones. If you then pile on more fiber, you are merely feeding the harmful microbes, making matters worse.

So, do not fill your diet with fiber-dense foods (such as beans, greens, fruits, and whole grains) if you have a severely unhealthy or unbalanced gut. With that caveat in mind, fiber is a crucial aspect of a gut-friendly diet. Ultimately when helpful microbes eat and ferment fiber, they produce Gut Gems.

Western Diet—High on PUFS, Low on Support for Gut Gems

The typical Western diet has created a complicated relationship to fiber in multiple ways. First, not much fiber exists in the foods many of us eat every day—whether that is pizza, pasta, sandwiches, bagels, or French fries. Remember that our ancestral diet was rich in fiber from a diversity of plant foods—roots, tubers, berries, fruits, nuts, and seeds. Every grain our ancestors ate was whole (and thus contained all its natural fiber). In other words, we evolved to flourish when eating fiber.

The lack of fiber in our modern diet weakens our population of good gut bacteria and tamps down the production of the Gut Gems that keeps our whole system in balance. On top of that, most go-to foods are made with seed oils, processed ingredients, and toxic additives that favor unfriendly bacteria.

When your beneficial gut bacteria are depleted or imbalanced, they can't break down fiber efficiently. As a result, fiber may sit longer in the colon and ferment in ways that favor gas-producing or inflammatory microbes, leading to bloating, cramping, or discomfort.

High-fructose sodas and desserts complicate the gut environment all the more. Like PUFS, refined fructose can disrupt your gut's microbial balance and set off a chain reaction where colonocytes are forced to scramble for Gut Gems. Over time, that can further lower your threshold for fiber tolerance. The solution is to stabilize the environment so your beneficial microbes and colonocytes can handle fiber gracefully and put it to good use.

Refined Fructose—A Hidden Disruptor

Every time you peel an orange or unwrap a candy bar, you prepare to take in simple sugars called glucose and fructose. While they may appear very similar, the two behave very differently in your body.

Glucose is the type of sugar your cells put to use for quick energy; it is rapidly absorbed by the bloodstream and travels to your muscles and brain. Fructose, meanwhile, heads straight for your liver, where it is turned into energy under normal circumstances. That said, our modern diet of sweetened beverages and sugary snacks probably has you consuming far more fructose than your liver can process at once.

Refined fructose—the kind found in soda, sweet tea, coffee drinks, and fruit juice—is one of the most troublesome forms of sugar. You'll also find it in processed snacks such as cookies, cakes, candy, and doughnuts. Unlike the natural sugar found in whole fruits, which come with fiber and protective plant compounds, refined fructose rushes through your system without offering your gut microbes anything useful.

Ingesting an abundance of refined fructose essentially starves your good bacteria, which means they make fewer Gut Gems. At the same time, it feeds your unfriendly bacteria, reducing your Gut Gem production even more.

Meanwhile, sugar spikes and crashes can make you crave quick fixes. You may then seek more sugar or reach for a pill to quell your appetite. The effect of sugar is especially subversive if you are also ingesting a fair bit of fiber when your gut is too weak to handle it. You may blame fiber for the bloat, but refined sugar could be exacerbating the imbalance, fueling the wrong microbes that ferment fiber into discomfort rather than beneficial by-products.

If you notice that fructose-filled drinks and snacks make your gut uncomfortable, consider cutting back or swapping them for a treat that relies on stable fats or minimal sweeteners. Dial down each offender in a measured way, and you will likely see your tolerance for fiber or occasional sweets improve exponentially. Over time, as your colonocytes ramp up Gut Gem production, you may find you can enjoy a sweet bite here and there without the side effects.

Gut Tolerance and Fiber Tracking Table

Date	Meal	Food Items	Estimated Fiber (g)	Digestive Response	PUFS v/ Toxins / Fructose Exposure
July 22 (Day 1)	Breakfast	Store-bought blueberry muffin, coffee with flavored creamer	2g	Mild bloating	Yes—PUFS in muffin oils, fructose in creamer
	Lunch	Turkey sandwich with mayo on white bread, bag of potato chips	3g	Gassy, slight cramping	Yes—seed oils in mayo & chips, refined ingredients
	Dinner	Grilled chicken, white rice, steamed green beans	5g	Normal	Low—green beans good; mild PUFS in marinade
	Snacks	Granola bar, apple	4g	Slight bloating after granola	Yes—PUFS/fructose in granola bar; apple is natural
Daily Total			14g	Overall: Mild discomfort	Moderate to high exposure from processed items

Fig. 15: Use a tracking table to identify which fiber-filled foods your body reacts to, and how.

Fiber Map—Assess Your Current Intake

If you would like to know how much fiber you can tolerate or where you stand on the fiber spectrum, keep track of your eating habits over a few days. Take note if you grabbed a ready-made muffin at breakfast, a sandwich at lunch, and possibly a starchy side such as French fries with dinner. No matter what, include everything and tally up a rough fiber count for each meal. Next, ask yourself how well your system tolerated your choices. Did you experience bloating? Did you sail through the day without any discomfort?

Also add a column for exposure to toxins, PUFS, and fructose. Was your muffin loaded with PUFS and refined fructose? Did your sandwich come with a sauce made from questionable oils? If your daily habits include lots of convenience foods, your total PUFS, toxins, and fructose tally could easily outweigh the fiber you are taking in. That information provides a good starting point in determining if your colonocytes have the environment they need to thrive.

Once you better understand your gut's balance, you can decide if it seems stable enough for a slow increase in fiber. If not, first strive to reduce toxins, fructose, and PUFS. The exercise is not to determine your perfect ratio right away. The objective is to gain an understanding of your gut's current capacity and then adjust your intake accordingly.

Gut Game—Fiber Versus Toxin Scorecard

If you are the competitive type, make this a game. Each day, track your "fiber points" and your "toxin points." Fiber points come from eating things that naturally provide roughage, like a handful of fresh produce. Toxin points come from PUFS, preservatives, plastics, and high-fructose corn syrup. Set a rule: Each day, aim to keep toxin points lower than your fiber points. If you manage that, your gut has a chance to adapt.

Do not stress if you start with more toxin points than fiber points. The idea is to chip away at the toxins—like PUFS-filled oils and refined fructose—while slowly nudging your fiber upward according to what your gut can handle. You can keep a simple log on your phone or a sticky note in your kitchen. (No need to overthink it!) And watch how you feel. If your gut rebels with every attempt to add fiber, you still may have too many PUFS, toxins, and/or refined fructose in your diet.

Toxin vs. Fiber Scorecard

Date	🌼 Toxin 🌼	Toxin Points	🌼 Fiber 🌼	Fiber Points
April 16	Chips, salad dressing made with soybean oil, plastic takeout container, sweetened iced tea	4	Raw kale, raw onions, chickpeas (in salad), apple (midmorning snack)	4

Fig. 16: Use this scorecard to track your intake of toxins and fiber each day. Aim to make your daily fiber points higher than your toxin points.

Fiber's Glory Comes After Healing

Fiber can be marvelous once your gut is ready. As we've been saying, however, don't force it on a broken system. If you've eaten more beans and greens and wondered why you felt worse instead of better, you get the message!

Focus first on letting your beneficial microbes restore themselves by eating fewer PUFS and cutting refined fructose out of your daily diet. Layer in stable fats that encourage, rather than suppress, Gut Gem production. Once you sense your internal environment is less volatile, you can introduce fiber in small increments and see how your body reacts.

Over time, you might find you're digesting foods you once feared or notice that a simple portion of fiber leaves you satisfied rather than gassy. That's the difference between mindless fiber loading—hoping it solves everything—and a gut-first strategy that sets you up for real, stable health from the inside out. Once your gut is healed, you won't have to think about the fiber paradox. Getting fiber from the foods you love will just be part of a balanced life.

———

Mara's Promotion at Work Brings Struggles and New, Terrible Cookies

At the Chicago Zoo offices, Mara's new morning workload was brutal—tight project deadlines and endless critiques from her superiors. It felt as though she was never good enough.

A stack of papers towered on her desk, high enough to make her sweat just thinking about it. Tension in her belly wound tighter all week, like a tight wire on a spool.

She swallowed hard and reached for the jar of oatmeal–chocolate chip cookies in her office. She knew stress sabotaged gut health just as much as poor food choices, but who cared? This was different. She was famished. She needed energy.

She pulled the oatmeal–chocolate chip cookie from the jar and admired it. She could see the chunks of chocolate and the grains of oatmeal. She took just a nibble. *Oh!* It was perfection.

The cookie settled in her gut, and at first she felt a lift—an uptick of energy. But then a swift crash and the familiar pain of cramps twisted her gut. *Too much fiber, too soon. Darn it!* she thought.

Mara sat there, hunched at her office desk, not only severely fatigued but also in pain. She wondered, *Great. Now how am I going to finish this project in time?* She wilted into her glass desk. *If only I could go home and snuggle my cat . . .*

Mara stared at her computer absently. Her eyes fell out of focus on the screen. She reviewed a data sheet not once, not twice, but three times before her mind finally snapped into place. *Ugh!* She gritted her teeth. She needed to stop fueling herself with sugar when she was stressed. She may have been tired before, but this was horrible.

CHAPTER 13

Dysbiosis—When the Wrong Microbes Take Over

You have probably had days when your gut was not on board with your diet. Maybe you felt bloated all afternoon or you dozed off after lunch. You may have blamed the reactions on stress or poor sleep when the real issue was deeper: dysbiosis.

Dysbiosis is a medical way of saying that the wrong bacteria have invaded your colon and left your system to suffer the aftermath. Key triggers to this kind of invasion are toxins: PUFS, chemicals such as pesticides and emulsifiers, and refined fructose. These modern-diet staples feed bad bacteria and damage colonocytes. Colonocytes, as mentioned, form the protective lining of your colon. Therefore, when they struggle, all kinds of unwanted particles can leak from your colon and into your bloodstream, where they trigger inflammation. On top of that, when the colonocytes weaken or die off, extra oxygen lingers in the colon, where it does not belong. The excess oxygen, in turn, kills the good bacteria and opens a path for harmful microbes to take over.

Why Oxygen—in the Right Places—Matters for Gut Health

Oxygen is an important part of gut health. Colonocytes burn Gut Gems as their primary energy source, and that process demands oxygen. Their consumption of oxygen is what keeps your colon free from oxygen (anaerobic). An anaerobic environment is essentially a haven for beneficial bacteria: they thrive, manage digestion, and keep the harmful microbes from running rampant.

If your colonocytes suffer ongoing assaults from toxins, over time, they become fatigued. Instead of burning Gut Gems and using up oxygen, they barely function. Not only does a weakened gut barrier allow particles to escape, but it also allows oxygen to seep in. Once the oxygen level becomes too high, beneficial low-oxygen microbes can no longer survive. If you've ever noticed bloating after the simplest meal, you might have a colon environment that is so high in oxygen that most beneficial microbes have died off.

Each time you choose a product full of PUFS, you risk fueling the process that damages your colonocytes. Add in processed fructose and toxins, and the gut environment becomes a free-for-all for harmful microbes.

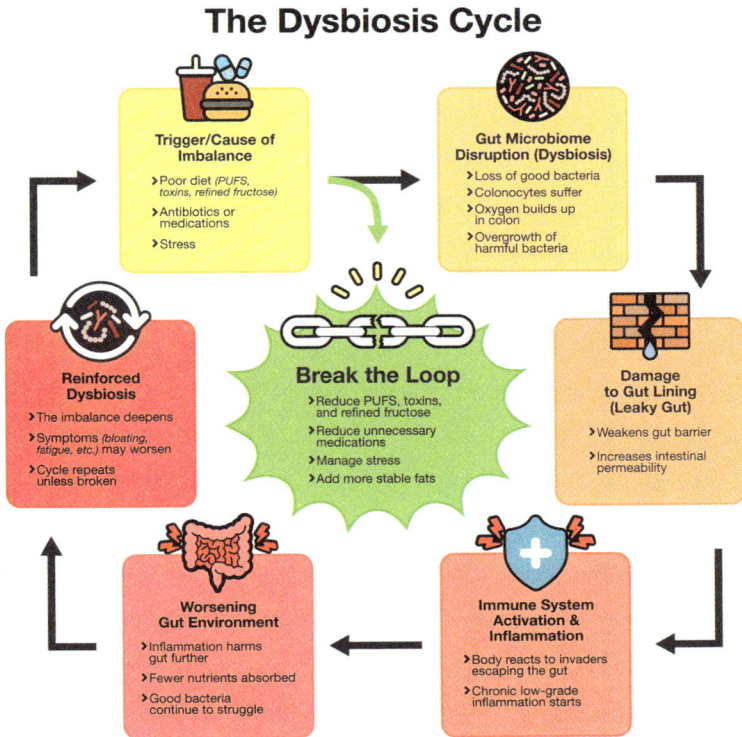

Fig. 17: Knowing the cycle of dysbiosis can help you break out of it.

In short, without a healthy population of colonocytes, your good gut bacteria lose the low-oxygen environment they rely on. That opens the door to dysbiosis. If the imbalance sticks around, it can throw off your whole system, triggering chronic inflammation, strange immune reactions, and a gut that never quite feels right.

Even worse, chronic issues such as autoimmune diseases, fatigue, skin problems, and mood disorders often take root when your immune system stays on high alert, triggered by molecules that should have been broken down and confined to the colon.

The fix involves clearing out the root cause—too many toxins that hamper colon cell function—so your system can stabilize. Once the colonocytes can burn Gut Gems properly, the likelihood of leaky gut or incessant inflammation decreases.

Dysbiosis Checklist—Identify and Conquer

Wondering if your gut is out of balance? Start by checking in with your body. Certain digestive patterns can offer clear clues about the state of your gut and whether it's time to take action.

Ask yourself the following:

1. Do you have a growing list of food intolerances? If you can only eat a limited number of foods without discomfort, it may be a sign your gut lining is compromised.

2. Do you feel bloated, gassy, or cramped after eating fiber-rich foods like fruit, potatoes, or vegetables? This can indicate trouble digesting key carbohydrates due to microbial imbalances.

3. Are your bathroom habits off? Ideally you should have at least one bowel movement per day. Going every other day—or less frequently—can signal sluggish digestion or inflammation.

4. Do you deal with chronic diarrhea or loose stools? Persistent bowel changes often point to irritation, inflammation, or poor microbial resilience.

Dysbiosis—When the Wrong Microbes Take Over

> If you answered yes to three or more of these questions, your gut is likely in a compromised state. Also consider how your daily habits may be fueling the problem. Are processed foods, refined sugar, or seed oils regular features on your plate? Are you exposed to pesticide residues from nonorganic produce or preservatives in snack foods? These factors chip away at your microbial defenses and help dysbiosis take root.
>
> Track your symptoms over the course of a week or two. Patterns will emerge. Do sugar cravings flare on days you eat more packaged snacks? Does your energy or mood dip after meals heavy in PUFS? By identifying the signs of dysbiosis early, you're setting yourself up for real, lasting change.

><

Mara Plans Meticulously and Realizes She's Too Uptight

Mara stood in her kitchen with her morning coffee and stared down at her food journal. After the fiasco at work with the cookie, Mara swore to be vigilant about reducing PUFS in her diet.

She rubbed her temples and jotted a few notes in the journal. The list of foods she once trusted was getting shorter, and each day brought greater challenges to avoiding PUFS.

Still, Mara was determined to solve the puzzle piece by piece. Not too long ago, she had learned that almonds had PUFS in them. A tiny amount of PUFS found naturally in an almond would usually be fine, but Mara's decades of overexposure meant she had to track everything. Write down everything. Mara sealed the bag of almonds and placed them in the freezer. She sliced a small wedge of cheese for her midafternoon snack instead.

At the gym, while walking on the stair machine together, Mara told Sarah that she's tracking everything—even the almond this morning.

Sarah shot her a questioning sideways glance.

"I know how it sounds," Mara blushed. "Like who tracks an almond, right?"

Sarah snapped her gaze back to the LED console to hide her reaction.

Mara felt a bit silly for admitting that she was tracking PUFS in an almond. "I just think once I get the hang of knowing what to eat, then I'll choose the right foods without thinking."

Sarah nodded. "Of course you will. And it's working. I never said you were uptight."

Later that night, Mara reclined on her bed. *Uptight. Uptight.* She petted the cat absently, and her mind wandered. Was she uptight? Now she couldn't get Sarah's voice out of her head!

She propped herself up on an elbow and read back through her journal. But she did notice the difference between prior days that were rife with bloating and fatigue and the changes over the past few days. Her tracking had helped!

>————◄

CHAPTER 14

Dysbiosis and Autoimmune Diseases

The immune system guards your body from intruders. All the same, it can harm your cells if it identifies them as potential threats. That is exactly what happens in certain autoimmune conditions. In other words, immune cells begin to attack the body's own tissues.

If your gut is full of harmful bacteria instead of beneficial ones, your immune system can react dramatically to the smallest irritation. The reason? The wrong microbes produce signals that stoke inflammation and push your immune system to see enemies everywhere, even in your own joints and organs.

When helpful microbes are plentiful, inflammatory signals drop because the immune system isn't looking to fight the body. The result is less joint pain and fewer flare-ups. If colonocytes are healthy, they consume Gut Gems and keep the oxygen in the colon low. A low-oxygen environment is ideal for beneficial microbes to flourish, without constant competition from harmful microbes. When your microbiome is in balance, the benefits go far beyond digestion. It's the difference between waking up with a body that is waging war on itself and one that is at peace.

How a Dysregulated Gut Leads to Dysregulated Immunity

Certain conditions such as rheumatoid arthritis, multiple sclerosis, and inflammatory bowel diseases (such as ulcerative colitis and

Crohn's) can make the immune system attack your own tissues. Such problems all track back to your gut. When colonocyte function is disrupted by dysbiosis or toxic foods, the gut barrier starts leaking, allowing proteins from food in the digestive tract to enter the bloodstream and trigger an immune response.

The immune system is remarkably intelligent. Nevertheless, it can be fooled. Proteins from partially digested food that slip through the gut barrier are larger than the smaller amino acids that would normally cross it. The immune system gears up to attack the larger proteins, but in doing so, it can also accidentally pursue similar-looking proteins in your joints (rheumatoid arthritis), nerve coverings (multiple sclerosis), and the intestines (ulcerative colitis, Crohn's). In medical research, autoimmunity is known as molecular mimicry for that very reason.

Medication might reduce symptoms, but it doesn't solve the deeper problem. Colonocytes are under siege. Therefore, they can't do their job of burning Gut Gems to keep the gut barrier sealed tight.

The good news is that if we can restore our colonocytes' ability to burn butyrate and use up oxygen in the process, we begin to reverse the conditions that cause leaky gut in the first place. Once beneficial microbes replace the harmful oxygen-dependent bacteria, the immune system senses less inflammation, so it stops damaging the body's own tissues. This effect pertains to all autoimmune conditions: Once the gut is calm, the immune system also calms.

Tregs to the Rescue

Tregs, or regulatory T cells, keep the immune system from overworking itself. Without enough Tregs, a minor trigger can spark various immune system responses. For example, joints can swell, nerve sheaths can fray, and intestines can become inflamed. Butyrate helps by nourishing colonocytes, and healthy colonocytes promote a gut environment that is hospitable to Tregs.

Tregs are the moderators that stop the immune system from punishing innocent bystanders (such as your joint linings or intestinal walls) for the slightest missteps. Increased Treg production calms everything down so there's less confusion and fewer flare-ups, so the body can heal.

Synergy between healthy colonocytes, stable microbe populations, and Treg expansion is the secret to preventing autoimmune conditions from spiraling out of control. So, when you come across any of the quick-fix solutions that promise miracles, remember that your body needs proper nourishment for Treg formation. A diet that is overloaded with PUFS degrades colonocytes and hampers Treg formation. Certain medications, such as NSAIDs, can also thin the gut barrier and worsen inflammation over time. Others, like immunosuppressants or steroids, may temporarily ease the symptoms, but it won't address the root issue in your gut. Therefore, your system will remain primed for rebellion.

How to Heal the Gut and Ease Autoimmune Struggles

To heal the gut, start by removing the PUFS that harm colonocytes. Once you do that, your cells can produce the Gut Gems needed to deplete oxygen in the colon and allow beneficial microbes to outcompete pathogens. Those good microbes, in turn, help lower inflammatory signals and foster Treg development, which keeps the immune system regulated.

Butyrate also has another way of reducing autoimmunity, particularly in rheumatoid arthritis, and that is by telling certain immune cells (T cells and macrophages) to calm down. Butyrate can further block signals such as NF-κB (nuclear factor kappa-light-chain-enhancer of activated B cells), which is a protein that promotes the production of inflammatory molecules such as cytokines. With a calmer immune system, the body is less likely to attack normal tissues.

The transition to a more regulated system is not instantaneous. Your body doesn't morph overnight. Instead, day by day, upon removing PUFS, refined fructose, and other toxins, as well as fueling your cells with stable fats, you can reduce the internal triggers that feed autoimmune conditions. Over time, fewer flare-ups will occur. If you've ever felt doomed by genetics or been told that you simply must "manage" your autoimmune condition, healing your gut might be the answer you've been waiting for.

Autoimmune Trigger Tracker

If you've been dealing with an autoimmune condition—anything from joint aches to odd skin reactions—it might help to track what you eat and how various foods make you feel. Besides jotting down what you put in your mouth and any symptoms you experience, also note other factors that seem to be influencing your body. Examples may include stress and poor sleep. Add a column to award yourself a point each time you are kind to yourself. That may mean eating a stable fat, avoiding refined fructose or other chemicals, or taking a walk to reduce your stress.

Keep the record for a couple of weeks and look for patterns. Do you find that your joints always seem to ache the day after you eat a deli sandwich with chips for lunch? Do you seem to concentrate better at work when you have a veggie omelet with good farmers market cheese for breakfast rather than toast and jam?

Over the course of a week or two, see how your system responds. Did you wake up without that random stiffness in your hands? Were your energy dips less dramatic? Pay attention to your body's feedback.

Mara and Sarah Have a Cooking Party to Help Sarah's Autoimmune Condition

Mara opened her front door for Sarah and pulled her in quickly from the cold autumn nighttime street.

"Thanks for hosting this party for me," Sarah flicked her blond hair over her shoulder in a flourish. "I love our new diet. I can't wait for the others to arrive." Sarah chewed Mara's sweet potato rolls before the party had even started. "This autoimmune nonsense is just something I've had since I was little," she blabbered. "My joints crack and ache, and I can even crack them so that they sing a song."

Mara's expression twisted and she stared at Sarah's knuckles briefly, then flicked her head away to the saucepan to keep herself from bursting out laughing. Mara stirred the potato crisps, then glanced back over her shoulder at her friend, who held her knuckles up to her ear.

"What surprised me most is how the dull ache in my joints faded." Sarah chewed a potato crisp. "My knees would feel hot and throb in the evenings, no matter how perfectly my deadlift had been, you know? I haven't noticed pain in my joints in weeks. It really is a reason to celebrate."

Sarah's miraculous recovery sent Mara digging into the details. She learned that food proteins can slip through a leaky gut and mimic the proteins in her own joint tissues. Mara thought, *I need evidence that PUFS in my diet might be a cause of my stiff knees.*

———

CHAPTER 15

When Your Gut Picks a Fight with Your Heart

Dysbiosis can spark fires of inflammation that blaze all the way to the heart. Your body is a complex network of pathways. When gut bacteria become imbalanced, the immune system goes on red alert and sends panic signals that spread from the digestive tract to the rest of the body. Your arteries can end up receiving a wave of signals that they interpret as a threat.

As you just learned, a balanced digestive tract fosters a calm immune system. In turn, the entire vascular system—the small and large pathways that carry blood—can operate without being stressed and always on alert. That basic understanding is important, but we also need to identify what causes the alarm bells to ring in the first place.

The Real Culprit Behind Heart Troubles: Oxidized LDL

You've probably heard that high LDL (low-density lipoprotein)—or "bad" cholesterol—is the main villain behind heart disease. But the real problem isn't LDL itself but rather what happens when LDL gets damaged. PUFS are highly unstable and break down easily when exposed to heat, light, or even just the oxygen inside your body. One of the by-products of that breakdown is reactive aldehydes—toxic molecules that attack your LDL particles. The result? Oxidized LDL.

Once oxidized, LDL no longer functions as a helpful delivery vehicle. Instead, your immune system targets it, triggering inflammation and setting the stage for plaque buildup in your arteries.

That's the true heart risk—not LDL per se but rather its damaged, oxidized version.

Yes, studies show a link between high LDL and heart disease. But dig deeper and you'll see it's not the quantity of LDL that matters— it's the quality. Your body actually needs LDL to transport nutrients and build hormones. What you don't need are the rogue by-products from PUFS that turn LDL toxic.

The fix isn't to cut out all fats—it's to cut the harmful ones. Removing PUFS and replacing them with stable fats such as butter, ghee, tallow, or coconut oil strengthens your LDL particles by making their membranes more resistant to oxidation. That means fewer opportunities for them to turn toxic, trigger inflammation, or fuel plaque buildup—giving your heart and gut a break from constant damage control.

The PUFS-Oxidized LDL Pathway: A Key Heart Risk

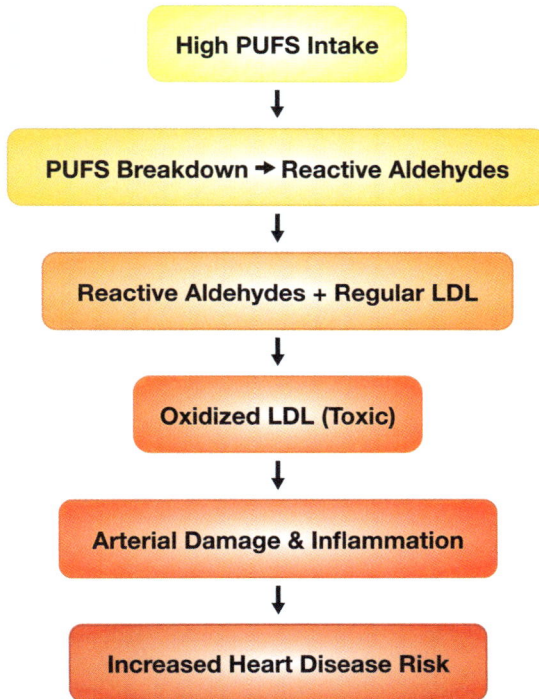

High PUFS Intake

↓

PUFS Breakdown → Reactive Aldehydes

↓

Reactive Aldehydes + Regular LDL

↓

Oxidized LDL (Toxic)

↓

Arterial Damage & Inflammation

↓

Increased Heart Disease Risk

Stable fats (butter, etc.) do not trigger this pathway

Fig. 18: Oxidized LDL increases heart disease risk, and PUFS contribute to its formation.

The Gut Gem–Heart Health Connection

Restoring harmony in the digestive tract means calling in Gut Gems. As we have discussed, those incredible compounds help reduce inflammation, protect your gut lining, and calm the immune system.

Butyrate helps reduce inflammation throughout the body—including in the arteries—by keeping the gut lining tight and preventing the release of toxins into the bloodstream where they can trigger an immune response. Butyrate also works with the immune system to dial down overactive responses. That means fewer unnecessary inflammatory attacks on the arteries.

Controlling inflammation is important. Once your bloodstream has recovered from inflammation, your heart can function more easily. Likewise, your vessels can do their work of carrying precious oxygen and nutrients instead of fending off inflammation.

Propionate and LDL: The Heart's New Best Friend

When health gurus chat about cholesterol, they often create a scary image that makes you afraid to eat eggs, butter, and other fats. However, the truth about cholesterol is far more nuanced than it's made out to be.

Your liver pumps out cholesterol because it is essential for hormone production, cell membranes, and a slew of vital processes. When your system is overloaded with stress, inflammation, or nutrient imbalances, the liver can go into overdrive, producing more very low-density lipoprotein (VLDL)—precursors to LDL particles—raising the amount of circulating LDL cholesterol.

This is when propionate—a Gut Gem that helps keep LDL levels from rising out of control—steps in. Propionate tells your liver, arteries, and immune cells to ease up on the cholesterol.

That said, propionate won't appear out of thin air. You need a healthy microbial environment in your gut that is capable of producing it. Restoring a balanced gut means giving that beneficial group of microbes the chance to flourish so they can churn out plenty of propionate and keep your LDL within healthy limits.

This method of working with your body's natural processes supports healthier cholesterol levels without the side effects of medications that can leave you feeling tired and sore. Another benefit of the natural approach is that you don't have to demonize real foods. You can enjoy butter and grass-fed steak *and* support your gut. Low-fat fads, in fact, deprive your body of what it needs.

Fiber Might Not Help Your Heart (Right Now)

Many experts suggest eating more fiber to protect your heart health. But there's a catch: Your gut might not be ready for fiber if it is still inflamed. Imagine trying to run a marathon when you've barely recovered from a twisted ankle. When the gut is less inflamed, you can gradually reintroduce fiber.

There's no one-size-fits-all timeline when it comes to adding fiber back into your diet. The best pace is the one your body agrees with. Start small and simple—think cooked veggies or a handful of fresh berries. Choose foods you actually enjoy so that the changes feel sustainable, not forced.

As for when to level up? Your gut will let you know. If your bloating has eased, and your bowel movements are regular and well-formed, that's a green light. It means your gut lining is stronger, your microbes are more balanced, and you're ready to handle a little more fiber. If instead you feel gassy, crampy, or sluggish after a fiber-rich meal, that's a sign to slow down and give your gut more time to heal.

Healing Dysbiosis for a Stronger Heart

Another way to rein in dysbiosis is to manage stress. Stress hormones such as cortisol and norepinephrine can shift the balance of your microbes, leaving you with an abundance of harmful bacteria and a lack of beneficial butyrate and propionate.

Stress also disrupts the mucus barrier, reduces intestinal blood flow, and impairs motility, all of which make your gut lining more vulnerable to inflammation and leaky gut. That permeability allows bacterial fragments, like lipopolysaccharides (LPS)—an endotoxin— to leak into circulation, triggering immune responses that affect your entire body, including your heart and brain.

This negative cycle highlights the importance of minding your emotional well-being. Whether you choose to take a slow walk around the block, dance to your favorite song, or practice a little grace and self-forgiveness, every bit helps.

As you gradually reclaim your gut's balance, beneficial Gut Gems will return. More butyrate and propionate mean less inflammation and steadier cholesterol numbers. Your arteries won't be bombarded by panic signals, and as a result, your heart's workload will lighten.

Why Quick-Fix Solutions Miss the Mark

Our culture loves a fast fix—especially one that doesn't ask you to change what's on your plate. But when it comes to heart health, quick-fix solutions such as cholesterol-lowering medications often miss the bigger picture.

Statins, for example, are among the most prescribed drugs for lowering LDL cholesterol. While they can reduce your numbers, they can also come with side effects—muscle pain, fatigue, brain fog, and even an increased risk of type 2 diabetes in some cases. And even when they seem to work, they may only be treating a symptom, not the source.

If your gut is inflamed and your microbiome is out of balance, your body continues to send out inflammatory signals. That means your arteries, joints, and tissues may still be under attack —even if your lab results show lower LDL. On paper, you look fine. But under the surface, the real problem is still smoldering.

That's why relying on medications alone can be misleading. If the gut lining is compromised, healing your heart isn't just about cholesterol—it's about calming the immune system, rebuilding the gut barrier, and restoring your body's ability to regulate inflammation.

Real healing takes time. It doesn't come in a bottle or with a slick advertisement. But when you nourish your gut and support your body's natural defenses, you give yourself a path to better heart health—without the drag of daily side effects or the illusion of a fix.

Your body is designed to heal. If you get a paper cut, you don't have to hover over it, chanting mantras to close the wound. Your skin naturally gets to work. Your gut is also capable of a remarkable bounce-back if given a chance.

After adjusting aspects of your lifestyle, you might discover that you're no longer winded walking up a hill. Your mood is brighter. Your skin is clearer. Your mind is sharper. That's what happens when your body's systems are not stuck in a cycle of fighting off the next crisis. They can finally channel energy to help you thrive, not merely survive.

So, if you ever catch yourself thinking you're doomed because your cholesterol numbers aren't picture-perfect, or you're worried about how some chest flutters might turn into something worse, remember this: You can support your heart by healing your gut.

Take a breath, give your body credit for making it this far. Move forward by diving into the real work of healing dysbiosis. Your body will reward you in ways you never thought possible.

―――――

Jake Has a Heart Issue at the Gym and Mara Attempts to Save His Life

Mara strode through the downtown Chicago gym greeting her friends before their morning workout. She wore the new pink leggings that Sarah had given her. She felt so confident in them. Mara caught sight of Jake at a treadmill across the way.

"Oh, Jake!" Mara waved him down.

Jake clutched his chest and stepped down from the treadmill. He looked winded, and his face was bright red.

"You all right?" Mara asked. Jake nodded and coughed.

"I got my annual labs back yesterday," Jake said, "and the results showed that my LDL cholesterol has shot above normal."

Mara nodded like she knew what that meant. But she did not.

Jake shrugged. "I knew that high LDL might lead to heart disease or stroke. But I'm working on making it better." He swatted a hand in the air. "It's nothing."

Mara tilted her head, unsure how to respond. Jake went to his friend across the room, and the moment passed.

That night at home, Mara whipped open her computer in a heated frenzy. *LDL, oh my gosh,* she thought. *I could save him. How amazing would that be? I have to research how to reduce LDL.*

Mara dove into a rabbit hole of information and learned that it's not necessarily how much LDL Jake has; it's damaged LDL or oxidized LDL. And how does LDL get damaged? When PUFS are digested, they break down into molecules called reactive aldehydes that interact with LDL, changing it into its evil cousin, oxidized LDL.

Mara slapped her laptop closed. *That's it!* she thought. *If Jake does this diet with me, I can save him.*

>———◄

CHAPTER 16

Akkermansia Repair and Reseeding: A Postbiotic to Probiotic Protocol

Colonocytes are tasked with keeping your gut lining tight so substances can't seep into your bloodstream. However, these cells are delicate and easily damaged if surrounded by PUFS or starved of Gut Gems, especially butyrate. In fact, colonocytes get about 70 percent of their energy from butyrate, while the other 30 percent comes from Gut Gems such as propionate and acetate.

That's why butyrate is the standout champion for fueling colonocytes. But if your gut is in chaos, the fastest way to recovery isn't pouring in butyrate from a bottle—it's repairing the lining and then reseeding the right microbes so your colon can make Gut Gems on its own. In chapter 3, I introduced this two-phase recovery strategy. Here, we'll take a deeper dive into the details of this protocol.

When to Start the Postbiotic to Probiotic *Akkermansia* Ramp

Begin Phase 1 whenever fiber "backfires," causing bloat, urgency, or cramping, or when barrier stress is obvious, resulting in things like food reactivity or flares. Postbiotic *Akkermansia*—pasteurized cells or their outer-membrane vesicles—delivers Amuc_1100 to the colon wall without feeding dysbiosis. After several weeks to a few months—whenever symptoms ease and stools and energy stabilize, transition into Phase 2: live *Akkermansia* plus *tolerable* prebiotics to rebuild the oxygen-poor, Gut Gem-producing community.

How to Choose *Akkermansia* Postbiotics (Phase 1) and Live *Akkermansia* (Phase 2)

Before we dive into specifics, it helps to understand the logic behind sequencing. Phase 1 starts with postbiotics—the stable, non-living parts of *Akkermansia* that can still deliver powerful proteins like Amuc_1100 that helps strengthen the tight junctions in the gut lining. Once that foundation is laid and the gut barrier has had time to strengthen, you can move on to Phase 2 with live *Akkermansia,* which needs a healthier environment to thrive. Think of it as rebuilding the house: you secure the walls first, then invite in the tenants.

- Choose *postbiotic* forms of *Akkermansia* (pasteurized whole cells or outer membrane vesicles) with enteric coating or microencapsulation that naturally protect Amuc_1100 until it reaches the colon.

- Why protection matters: If you swallow *naked* Amuc_1100 (no enteric coating), by the time it reaches the colon, less than 5 percent may remain.

- Workarounds: You could try to "dose around" this by taking a 100-times greater dose, but that's expensive and imprecise. For best results, prioritize protected formats.

- When ready, add *live* (probiotic) *Akkermansia*, paired with small doses of well-tolerated prebiotics to feed butyrate-producers without reigniting bloat.

- Remember the goal: you're rebuilding the low-oxygen ecosystem that powers most of your Gut Gem supply—*Akkermansia* plus its obligate-anaerobe (oxygen-sensitive) partners.

Keep Your Diet Clean When Adding Supplements

Postbiotics aren't magic wands. The gut barrier is still sensitive while healing. Keep PUFS out, keep stress to a minimum, and keep meals simple while the lining repairs. The calmer the terrain, the faster Amuc_1100's "tighten and heal" message takes hold, and the smoother your transition to live *Akkermansia* and your body's natural production of Gut Gems like butyrate.

A Practical Two-Phase Protocol (Low and Slow)

Phase 1—Repair using enteric coated/microencapsulated postbiotic *Akkermansia*. Remember, if protected formats are not available and you must use an unprotected product, expect to lose up to 95 percent of the Amuc_1100 during transit.

- Week 1: Take a small daily dose (the product's lowest serving) with a simple meal; assess how you feel at 48–72 hours.

- Weeks 2–4: Increase to the standard daily dose if you have no bloating or urgency.

- Weeks 4–12: Maintain the standard dose while you simplify meals (low PUFS, low emulsifiers), walking daily and prioritizing sleep. Watch for signals of repair: fewer food reactions, calmer stools, steadier afternoons.

Phase 2—Reseed with probiotic (live) *Akkermansia* plus gentle, well-tolerated prebiotics.

- Add live *Akkermansia* while continuing the postbiotic for 2–4 more weeks.

- Introduce small doses of well tolerated prebiotic foods, such as a spoonful of cooked-and-cooled rice or potato or a few bites of green-banana flour in yogurt.

- Expand the variety of prebiotic inputs every week or two as comfort allows. The goal is to have no flares while beneficial bacteria repopulate and Gut Gems rise.

- If bloat returns, pause prebiotics for three to five days; maintain postbiotic and live *Akkermansia*, then try reintroducing prebiotic foods again at half the previous amount.

At some point, you may end up asking, "How do I know if any of this is really working?" The answer comes from paying attention to subtle signals from your body and trusting the cumulative effect of the changes. Does your digestion feel smoother? Are your energy levels consistent throughout the day? If the changes are real, you will know it.

For a tangible way to track progress, write a few lines each day about how you feel physically and mentally. A quick note in your phone is sufficient. Record when you take your postbiotic or live *Akkermansia* (morning versus night, with meals versus without) and note any changes in bloating or overall comfort. Over time, your notes will reveal patterns that show you where you are in the gut-healing process.

Remember, your body has its own timeline for rebuilding, and this repair and reseeding strategy merely guides that process along more smoothly. You will benefit more if you avoid fixating on every minor setback. Instead, view each new day as an opportunity to take another step in the right direction.

Reclaim Your Gut, Reclaim Your Life

Your gut is central to your day-to-day experience. If you're dealing with stubborn bloating, unpredictable bowel habits, or low energy, your ability to focus on the bigger joys becomes challenging. By zeroing in on strategies that heal your gut, you free yourself to live more fully. Imagine waking up with a calm belly and a clear mind—ready to take on the day without the usual sluggishness or second-guessing your breakfast. Picture running errands, going to work, or meeting friends without worrying whether your digestion will derail your plans.

That's the power of a healthy gut. When your gut is in balance, everything else—your focus, your energy, even your mood—starts to follow suit. It becomes easier to show up for your work, your relationships, and your downtime with more ease and less stress. In short, restoring your gut isn't just about improving digestion—it's about creating a steady foundation for your entire life.

That said, remember that healing your gut is rarely a straight line from point A to point B. You'll have detours with moments of self-doubt and times that you cave to familiar temptations. The goal is not to chase perfection but to cultivate an overall resilient gut.

Phase 1 gives your lining breathing room; phase 2 hands the job back to your microbes. Postbiotics help you bounce back faster from occasional missteps; live *Akkermansia* and gentle prebiotics lock in the win by restoring the community that makes Gut Gems naturally. As you refine your relationship with food—especially your avoidance of PUFS—you lay the groundwork for a life that isn't dominated by digestive drama.

Will you need *Akkermansia* supplements forever? Probably not. Most people keep a small postbiotic "safety net" during stressful seasons or travel, then rely on fermented foods they tolerate, and a low-PUFS diet to maintain the ecosystem that cranks out Gut Gems. If your history includes frequent digestive flares, you may want to use a low maintenance dose of postbiotic *Akkermansia* longer than 12 weeks, and that's perfectly fine. Just taper it as your gut's resilience returns.

>———◀

Mara Takes a Chill Pill

At home with her afternoon mint tea, Mara scrolled through internet articles and supplement factoid pages, desperate to find a supplement to support her gut. After listening to one of Dr. Ellis's lectures, Mara became convinced she needed a probiotic supplement, specifically. She chewed her lip, searching. *It makes sense that they could help reseed the microbiome and support my mood* she thought. Taking a probiotic would also provide backup; in case she mistakenly ate something with PUFS, her gut lining would hopefully be stronger. Mara picked out a special enteric coated probiotic supplement so that it would survive the trip through her digestive system. She ordered a bottle and was delighted when the package arrived at her door. She worked the supplement into her routine, taking it with dinner.

Mara recorded how much she took, when she took it, and how her digestion responded in her special food journal. She was astonished that it only took a few days to get positive results.

One night, Sarah texted: You seem so chill lately—what's your secret?

Mara smiled and typed back: I took a chill pill.

Sarah wrote: Huh?

Mara wrote: It's this new probiotic supplement I'm taking. I'll show you next time we meet.

———

CHAPTER 17

Probiotics: Rebuild Your Gut with Friendly Microbes

Let's say you're sitting at your kitchen table, looking at three different probiotic bottles. Each one promises to rescue your gut, fill you with energy, and help you look ten years younger. You also have a carton of yogurt in the fridge, a jar of kimchi, and some sauerkraut that has been skulking on the back shelf for who knows how long.

You're probably wondering if you need any of it. The short answer: Yes. Probiotics are friendly bacteria that can help your digestive system, especially when you choose strains that naturally boost your production of Gut Gems. Think of beneficial microbes such as *Bifidobacteria* or *Lactobacillus* as your new allies. You want them around because they produce beneficial by-products that nourish your colonocytes, reduce inflammation, and create calmness in the gut. Other lesser known but equally helpful microbes also thrive on specific compounds in your gut and turn them into extra nourishment for your cells.

Strains That Boost Gut Gem Production

If you're curious about why particular strains matter, the answer is that they help you produce plenty of Gut Gems like butyrate. Some strains appear in cultured foods such as yogurt, kefir, kimchi, and sauerkraut. Others can show up in well-formulated probiotic supplements. Be aware, however, that not every yogurt or probiotic brand contains the valuable strains.

Some products add in a couple of odd strains, and that's all. If you're in serious need of bolstering your Gut Gem production, choose foods or supplements known to harbor some of the most powerful strains like *Bifidobacterium*, *Lactobacillus*, and some of the more exotic ones you'll learn about in this chapter. Also keep in mind that not all fermented foods deliver live microbes—pickles made with vinegar, for example, may be sterile. Look for labels that say "raw" or "unpasteurized" to ensure the microbes are still active.

Probiotics, Butyrate, and a Harmonious Gut

Probiotic supplements supply beneficial microbes to the gut so it can create more Gut Gems, including butyrate. Also, when colonocytes are fueled by enough Gut Gems, they can plug any leaks in your gut lining. In other words, particles are not seeping into the bloodstream and firing up your immune system. As a result, you'll have less chronic inflammation. The ripple effect includes an improvement in everything from your joint comfort to your mental clarity.

Probiotics can also create more energy and fewer sugar cravings. The reason? Your gut has a direct line of communication with your brain. When your gut is balanced, your brain usually is too. In short, probiotic supplements help support your entire body, especially if your gut was previously burdened under the weight of too many PUFS and processed foods.

Behind the Scenes of Your New Gut Crew

Let's examine the lesser-known strains in your probiotic arsenal, which are often overshadowed by big names like *Lactobacillus* or *Bifidobacterium*.

Some of these unsung heroes include:

- *Akkermansia muciniphila*
- *Anaerobutyricum hallii* (formerly *Eubacterium hallii*)
- *Anaerostipes spp.*
- *Clostridium kluyveri*
- *Clostridium leptum*

- *Eubacterium rectale*
- *Faecalibacterium prausnitzii* (also known as *Faecalibacterium duncaniae*)
- *Lachnospira eligens*
- *Phocaeicola vulgatus* (a reclassified genus formerly under *Bacteroides*)
- *Roseburia intestinalis*

These bacteria are specialists in producing or promoting Gut Gems. If you find a supplement that contains one or more of these in a stable, oxygen-protected form, it might be extremely helpful.

However, the fact that a bacterium is listed on the label doesn't necessarily mean you'll get enough living microbes to make a difference. Always keep an eye out for how the product is made. Did the manufacturer mention anything about oxygen-free packaging? How about enteric coated or time-release capsules? Does the label say "50 billion CFUs" without explaining how they are kept alive? A high quantity is meaningless if the majority die before they enter the colon.

Only if the strains mentioned enter the gut alive can they establish themselves and contribute to a healthier gut environment. The possibility exists that certain strains will click better with you than others. That's normal. As we've said, your microbiome is unique, shaped by everything from birth circumstances to antibiotic history. The best approach is to start with a good-quality product, track how you feel for a few weeks, and then decide if you need to adjust anything.

Probiotics and Oxygen Sensitivity: Why Delivery Matters

Many of the best strains of gut bacteria hate oxygen. That creates a challenge. Why? The small intestine is loaded with oxygen, while the colon is largely oxygen-free.

If your probiotic supplements dissolve before they reach the colon—which is where these fragile microbes really belong—they will be ineffective. They'll encounter too much oxygen in the small intestine and be destroyed long before they can do any good.

Some newly developed probiotic products now use specialized, microencapsulated delayed-release tablets designed to protect oxygen-sensitive microbes so they don't dissolve in the oxygen-rich small intestine. By insulating the microbes until they reach the lower parts of your digestive tract, the capsules ensure that the fragile microbes arrive alive to do their job.

The details of release in a capsule are vital and big news if you have tried probiotics and felt no difference. The microbes never had a fighting chance to survive where they were needed. Moving forward, when you're shopping for a new probiotic supplement, pay attention to any mention of delayed release or colon-targeted delivery. If you don't see that promise, there's a chance you'll end up disappointed.

The same is true for oxygen exposure during manufacturing. Some of the lesser-known strains—such as *Akkermansia muciniphila* or *Faecalibacterium prausnitzii*—are extremely oxygen-sensitive. Therefore, if the manufacturer failed to handle them with care, the strains could be dead by the time you open the bottle. This is a prime reason to be picky in sourcing your probiotic. You may pay a little more, but you're investing in living organisms that need the right conditions to survive.

All things considered, real-food options deliver advantages. Foods such as kimchi and sauerkraut create an anaerobic environment as they ferment. That's why they emit a tangy aroma: Beneficial microbes are feeding on the sugars in the vegetables and multiplying in an oxygen-limited setting. Also, you get the bonus of other nutrients that are not present in a supplement.

Probiotic Matchmaker

All the strains of probiotics available can cause confusion. Which ones should you seek? The following chart lists the unique benefits of several known probiotic strains to help you prioritize the options

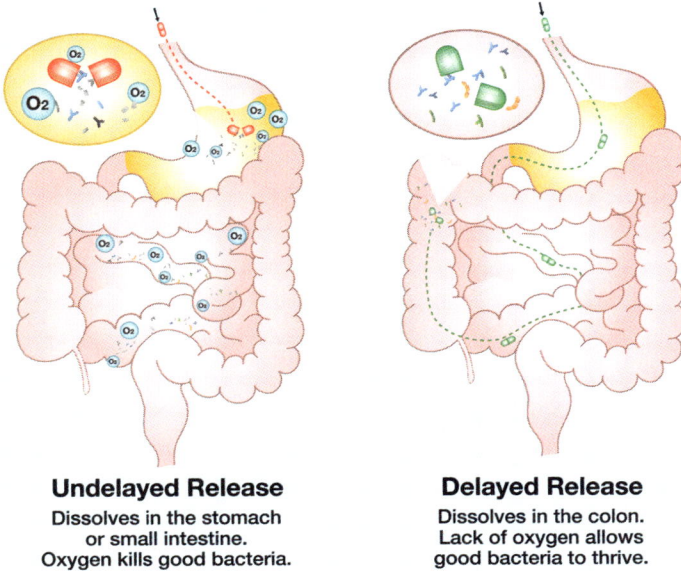

The Role of Formulation in Probiotic Effectiveness

Undelayed Release
Dissolves in the stomach
or small intestine.
Oxygen kills good bacteria.

Delayed Release
Dissolves in the colon.
Lack of oxygen allows
good bacteria to thrive.

Fig. 19: When probiotic supplements break down too soon, the oxygen-sensitive bacteria they contain die before reaching the colon, where Gut Gems are produced.

when you shop for supplements. While the table is based on current scientific research, effects can vary from person to person. The only way to learn what's best for you is to experiment. In the process, take note of how you feel after trying each strain.

When Fermented Foods Are Your Friend (and When They're Not)

Fermented foods can be a lifesaver once your gut is stable. If your digestive system is still healing, they can sometimes trigger a storm. Picture your gut as a building site under repair. Too many lively microbes arriving all at once is like having an amped-up construction crew show up before the scaffolding is set. No one can work, so everyone is anxiously pacing, getting in each other's way.

Probiotics Types

Probiotic Strain	Helps With
Bifidobacterium	Constipation, gas, and boosting good gut bacteria
Lactobacillus	Diarrhea, bloating, and supporting the immune system
Akkermansia muciniphila	Weight management and blood sugar control
Faecalibacterium prausnitzii	Calming gut inflammation and easing IBS symptoms
Phocaeicola vulgatus	Reducing gut inflammation and improving gut balance
Roseburia intestinalis	Improving bowel movements and reducing belly pain
Agathobacter rectalis	Making butyrate (a gut-healing fuel) and reducing gas
Faecalibacterium duncaniae	Easing inflammation and protecting gut lining
Segatella copri	Breaking down fiber and helping control blood sugar
Alistipes shahii	Supporting a healthy gut and easing gut irritation
Barnesiella intestinihominis	Helping prevent harmful bacteria from growing
Lachnospira eligens	Supporting digestion and healthy immune response
Dorea formicigenerans	Assisting digestion and reducing harmful bacteria
Clostridium leptum	Producing butyrate and calming gut inflammation
Oxalobacter formigenes	Helping prevent kidney stones by breaking down oxalates

Fig. 20: While you don't need every single strain of probiotics, the more diverse your microbiome is, the more resilient it is.

Without a strong gut lining, too much fermented food can leave you bloated or running to the bathroom. Proper timing is key for introducing probiotics. If you've recently eliminated PUFS, and your stomach feels calmer, you might be ready for some probiotics. Consider yogurt, kefir, or a small portion of sauerkraut.

In contrast, if your gut remains sensitive, and simple meals still cause discomfort, proceed cautiously or wait. Adding a large amount of kimchi or other fermented foods could overwhelm your system. Start with small portions, monitor your body's response, and gradually increase only when your gut signals it's ready.

Also, consider your tolerance for dairy if you're aiming for yogurt or kefir. Some people handle it fine. Others find it sets off bloating or skin issues. If the latter is the case, you might handle kimchi or sauerkraut better, which are made with cabbage and other vegetables.

Use portion size as your safety net. For example, start with only a spoonful of kimchi. See how you feel a few hours later or the next day. If you did not encounter any problems, try a bit more next time. If you experienced discomfort, scale back.

Keep PUFS Out of the Picture

If you're taking probiotics but still eating PUFS-filled foods, you may as well try to fill a bucket that has a giant hole. No matter how many beneficial bacteria you pour in, the environment will remain inflammatory and the delicate strains will not flourish. Sure, some might manage to cling on and help a little, but you'll never feel the full benefit.

Cutting back on PUFS is a crucial step. At the same time, feed your gut the saturated fats we have recommended. Once you've lowered the inflammation in your gut, your newly introduced microbes will have a solid foothold to begin producing Gut Gems. As your colonocytes receive ample fuel, they use it to rebuild and keep your gut lining sealed, setting in motion a positive feedback loop.

Learn to Trust Your Gut Again

After months (or years) of dealing with gut issues, you might have lost faith in your body. Maybe you've been living with the possibility that something you eat could trigger a mini anxiety attack. Perhaps you've been skipping social events because you never know how your belly will behave. Reintroducing probiotics can help you regain trust in your digestion.

You may also notice changes in your mood and energy thanks to the gut-brain connection. When your microbial population starts producing beneficial compounds, and when your gut lining is intact, your entire system calms.

Of course, you can still have days when things aren't great. Stress, travel, or an encounter with a PUFS-loaded snack can trigger little setbacks. Overall, however, with a sturdier baseline, your body will be more resilient.

Expand Your Microbial Horizons

Once your gut is stable enough to explore new foods, you can be more adventurous with fermented goodies. Each type of fermentation introduces different friendly bacteria, giving your gut a broader range of microbial allies.

Always remember to check in with your body's response. A moderate approach, gradually introducing new strains or fermented dishes, often yields the best results. And if you ever find yourself feeling overwhelmed, take a small step back. Healing is a dynamic process, not a straight line to the finish.

You might also stumble upon new probiotic formulas that claim to have the most cutting-edge strains on the market. Some might genuinely colonize your gut and produce helpful by-products. Others might not be worth the money. Read the labels carefully, look for those that mention time-release or colon-targeted technology, and keep an eye out for oxygen-sensitive packaging. If you're going to invest in probiotics, you want to be sure you're buying living microbes that can survive the gastrointestinal tract to reach their intended destination.

Just remember, real food remains your long-term best friend. Supplements can bridge gaps, especially if you're coming from a place of severe imbalance. Eventually, though, you want to rely on nutritious meals that properly feed your cells. When your gut has consistent support from real food, it tends to reward you with a calmer, more vibrant life.

Four-Week Good Microbes Adventure

Although gut health is nothing to laugh at, you can—and should— have fun while working to improve it. Let's try a good-microbes adventure. Your mission: to mix it up, maintain a sense of playfulness and curiosity, and let your gut throw a "good-microbes party" every week!

Four-Week Good Microbes Adventure

Week	Good Microbe Focus	Try This	Fun Bonus Tip
1	*Lactobacillus*	Yogurt with live cultures, kefir, or a probiotic supplement	Add berries and a dash of honey to yogurt for dessert!
2	*Bifidobacterium*	Probiotic supplement, miso soup, or sauerkraut	Heat miso to warm (not boiling) to keep microbes alive.
3	*Faecalibacterium* boosters	Eat high-fiber foods (beans, oats, bananas) to help these microbes grow	If your gut is still recovering, start with a very small portion—even a tablespoon or two.
4	*Akkermansia* boosters	Take a supplement or eat pomegranate and cranberries and drink green tea	Sip iced green tea with lemon in the afternoon.

Fig. 21: The more diverse your microbiome is, the more resilient it is. Boost diversity by focusing on a different microbe each week.

Each week, pause to ask yourself:

- How is my digestion?
- Am I feeling more energized or lighter?
- What digestive changes do I notice? Do I have less bloating? Am I more regular?

Carving Your Own Path Toward Microbiota Restoration

Your gut is as unique as your thumbprint, shaped by your diet history, antibiotic use, stress levels, and a variation of life factors that might not affect anyone else. That means no published guidelines can tell you exactly which strains or how many billion CFUs you need. Instead, think of this chapter as a road map that highlights major landmarks with the recommendation to proceed slowly. Once your gut settles down, you can move forward with more confidence. If *Bifidobacterium* helps you feel amazing, great. If a lesser-known microbe does wonders for your mood, that is a sign your microbiome is tuning in to your personal needs. Pay attention to how different parts of your body feel along the way.

Based on your reactions, you might choose to rotate probiotic sources, trying different foods or supplements every couple of months to keep your microbial ecosystem diverse. Some folks find that certain times of year—such as winter, when stress can run high—call for a bit more probiotic support. The key is staying flexible. This is not a strict prescription. You can and possibly should deviate from time to time.

><

Mara Eats Kimchi at Her Cousin's Korean Restaurant

Mara stationed herself at her kitchen table with a mug of green tea and devoted her Sunday afternoon to researching different probiotic supplements, some of which boasted like ten billion CFU (whatever that was). Interestingly enough, she learned that certain fermented foods have probiotics in them already. Foods like kimchi and sauerkraut. Both of them also contain prebiotic fiber that feed the good guys in the gut. That seemed like a good way to start.

After so many positive results taking her probiotic supplement, next on the list was investigating probiotics in foods. Apparently, both pre- and probiotic foods should be introduced once the gut barrier is healthy and the gut is fairly good to go.

That night, her family gathered at her cousin's Korean restaurant in downtown Chicago. Everyone sat crammed side by side at a long table, celebrating her nephew's graduation from middle school. Aunt Linda ordered bibimbap, rice, fish, tempura. Among the long list of sides included for the table was kimchi.

Oh my gosh, it's a sign, Mara thought. *I was just thinking about kimchi for the probiotics.* She craned her neck over to the waiter and ordered an extra side of kimchi for herself.

I'm going to try fermented foods again. My gut must be ready, she thought. She had come a long way since last year's ill-fated kimchi experiment when, after devouring half a jar while watching the latest action movie with a wildly charming movie star, she spent the next day stuck at home in a state of bloated misery.

Mara and her family ate and had animated conversation, and the food tasted delicious. She devoured her fish and kimchi, got swept up in family drama with Aunt Linda's memory issues, and hardly noticed the state of her gut.

Hours later, back at home in her fluffy slippers, Mara shuffled around the house humming a sweet song. She smiled at the cat. "It's working."

><

CHAPTER 18

Prebiotics and Dietary Strategies

Because prebiotics are not rapidly broken down and absorbed as glucose in the bloodstream, they do not cause quick spikes in blood sugar. Instead, they are fermented slowly by gut microbes, which is why they can be considered "slow-burn" carbs. Unlike *pro*biotic supplements, which add microbes, *pre*biotic food and supplements nourish the good bacteria already living in your gut. Your good gut microbes love prebiotics, which deliver fuel they need to produce essential Gut Gems and calm any inflammation underway in your cells. Therefore, prebiotics strengthen your microbiome over time.

Think of prebiotics as rich soil that helps your internal ecosystem grow strong and diversify. As you introduce prebiotic foods, start slowly and intentionally. Especially if your gut is sensitive, adding too much too quickly can lead to bloating and discomfort. Ideally begin with small portions, rotate your sources, and allow your microbiome to adjust gradually.

In a supplementation regimen, prebiotics can be considered after you've strengthened the tight junctions with postbiotic *Akkermansia* and then gradually introduced more good gut microbes by taking *Akkermansia* and other probiotics. Crucially, your gut should be feeling good with no regular bloating, constipation, or diarrhea.

Specific prebiotics include inulin, fructooligosaccharides (FOS), and galactooligosaccharides (GOS)—long strings of sugars that humans can't digest. This means prebiotics travel all the way to the colon intact. Once they reach the colon, *Bifidobacteria* and other friendly strains break them down. During that breakdown, the bacteria release Gut Gems that get to work thickening the mucus that protects your gut lining, seal up any microcracks in your gut wall, and remind your immune cells to keep calm.

Prebiotic Pathway

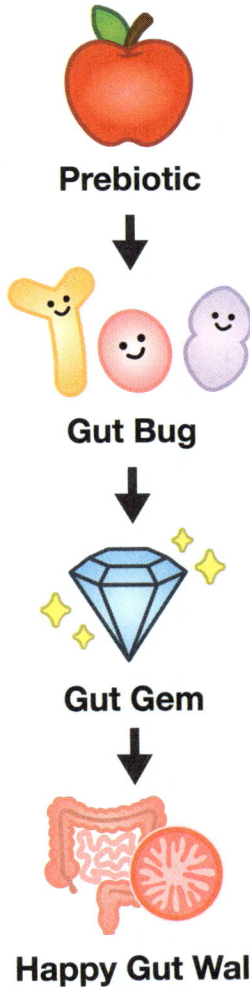

Prebiotic

Gut Bug

Gut Gem

Happy Gut Wall

Fig. 22: Eating prebiotics helps your good gut bugs thrive and produce plenty of Gut Gems, which then help strengthen the lining of your gut.

How to Add Prebiotics to Your Routine

Prebiotic fibers serve as food for beneficial gut microbes and can improve digestive comfort and immune resilience. Choose any of the following options to see which one fits your taste and tolerance best.

- **Inulin** comes from long chicory-root fibers that taste faintly sweet, dissolve nicely, and serve bakers who want to reduce the total sugar they use. Available in powder form, inulin is easy to incorporate in recipes. Just be sure to pair it with adequate fluids—especially water or broth—to help it move smoothly through your system and reduce the risk of constipation.

- **GOS,** occuring naturally in dairy, are beloved by *Bifidobacteria* and strains linked to clearer skin and tougher lung defenses.

- **FOS,** found in bananas, garlic, Jerusalem artichokes, and onions, are fast-acting fuel for *Lactobacilli*.

You can mix and match the different fibers. For example, on Monday you could stir half a teaspoon of inulin in your coffee and then wait twenty-four hours. If you had any bloat, cramps, or urgent bathroom breaks, you could pause, sip bone broth, and wait another day. If you felt fine on Tuesday, you could try a bit of GOS-rich yogurt for breakfast. On Wednesday, you might have some roasted garlic (prepared by drizzling butter over the bulb before wrapping it in foil) with dinner.

A deliberate drip-feed of prebiotics does two clever things. First, it trains your resident microbes to gear up enzyme production without staging a revolt. Second, it lets you map your personal tolerance curve before your gut becomes unpredictable.

Research shows that a 20-gram daily inulin dose can raise fecal Gut Gem levels by 25 percent in two weeks. That said, you don't want to race there on day one. Prebiotics are forms of fiber, and we've been discussing the need to reduce fiber as your gut heals and grows stronger. Therefore, don't aim to eat three bananas at once. Instead, test-drive tiny doses, listen for grumbles, then inch up only when the coast is clear. Some people have an increased sensitivity to certain foods that more easily ferment in the gut. This group may need even smaller doses to avoid problematic reactions.

Prebiotic Foods: Feed Your Gut the Right Way

Food	Key Prebiotic Compound	How to Eat It
Garlic	Inulin, Fructooligosaccharides (FOS)	Mince raw into dressings or mash into avocado; sauté in olive oil for stews; drizzle with butter and roast until soft.
Onions (especially raw)	Inulin, FOS	Add to salads, salsas, or slice into sandwiches; caramelize for gut-friendly sweetness.
Leeks	Inulin	Use in soups, frittatas, or roasted with root vegetables.
Asparagus	Inulin	Steam lightly, roast, or chop into warm grain bowls.
Jerusalem Artichokes	Inulin	Roast or slice thinly for salads; try pureed in soups.
Bananas (slightly green)	Resistant starch, Pectin	Slice into smoothies or blend with nut butter for a prebiotic-rich snack.
Chicory Root	Inulin	Brew as a coffee alternative or add chicory powder to smoothies.
Dandelion Greens	Inulin, FOS	Toss into salads, sauté with garlic, or blend into green smoothies.
Legumes (lentils, chickpeas, beans)	Galactooligosaccharides (GOS)	Add to soups, make hummus, or toss into salads.

Fig. 23: Use this chart as inspiration for adding more prebiotic foods to your diet as your gut can handle them. Remember, start small and monitor your symptoms before increasing your intake.

Gut-Brain Chatter: How Gut Gems Turn into Feel-Good Signals

Ever notice how a good meal can shift your mood? That's your gut-brain highway getting the green light from Gut Gems. Gut Gems slip through the colon lining, enter the bloodstream, and bind to receptors on your vagus nerve—the line of communication between your gut and your brain. The vagus nerve reads the situation in your gut and transmits signals that modulate mood and stress responses.

More specifically, Gut Gems bind to G-protein receptors on entero-endocrine cells (hormone-making tiles in your gut wall). Those cells release peptide hormones that signal everything is okay. Your brain receives the signal, drops cortisol, and loops in dopamine for a light hit of "Everything's fine." The result is steady energy, not a spike-and-crash.

Personalize Your Prebiotic Plan

If dairy upsets your stomach, consider GOS powder instead of GOS yogurt. GOS powder can be purchased online. It's also available through some health foods stores. If you are lactose intolerant, don't worry. Lactase drops plus aged Gouda can keep your prebiotic tank filled.

Another great prebiotic option is hazelnut muffins, sweetened with inulin and baked in butter. (See the following recipe). They are easy to make in large batches that you can store in the freezer and grab and enjoy on the go as part of your breakfast. Besides being tasty and satisfying your hunger for hours, each bite triggers a bump in Gut Gems that can last well past lunch and ward off snack cravings. If you're more concerned with maintaining your focus through afternoon assignments and meetings, have your inulin dose at lunchtime instead. A Gut Gem surge will land right when your brain usually hits the snooze button.

If your main goal is muscle repair, aim for 5 grams of GOS right after workouts. The Gut Gems should arrive just in time to lower exercise-induced inflammation. If smoother digestion is of utmost importance, pair roasted chicory root with peppermint tea at night. The combo eases spasms while feeding beneficial microbes.

Dr. Mercola's Prebiotic Hazelnut Muffins
Yield: Makes 12 muffins

Dry Ingredients
1½ cups hazelnut flour (prebiotic-rich, nutty flavor)
½ cup almond flour (for texture)
¼ cup inulin powder (prebiotic sweetener; feeds gut bacteria)
1 tsp baking powder
½ tsp baking soda
¼ tsp salt
1 tsp ground cinnamon (optional, for warmth)

Wet Ingredients

½ cup unsalted butter, melted (plus extra for greasing)

3 large eggs

⅓ cup milk

1 tsp pure vanilla extract

2 tbsp maple syrup (optional, for slight sweetness boost)

Add-Ins (optional)

⅓ cup chopped hazelnuts (for crunch)

¼ cup dark chocolate chips (85 percent cocoa or darker, low sugar)

Preheat oven. Set to 350°F (175°C). Grease a 12-cup muffin tin generously with butter or line with parchment liners.

Mix dry ingredients. In a large bowl, whisk hazelnut flour, almond flour, inulin powder, baking powder, baking soda, salt, and cinnamon (optional).

Combine wet ingredients. In another bowl, whisk melted butter, eggs, milk, vanilla extract, and maple syrup (optional) until smooth.

Combine wet and dry ingredients. Pour wet ingredients into the dry. Stir gently until just combined. Fold in chopped hazelnuts or chocolate chips or a blend of both (optional).

Fill muffin tin. Divide batter evenly among the 12 muffin cups (about ¾ full).

Bake. Bake for 18–22 minutes or until a toothpick comes out clean and tops are golden. Let cool in the tin for 5 minutes, then transfer to a wire rack to cool completely.

Freeze for storage. Once cooled, place muffins in a single layer in a freezer-safe bag or container. Freeze for up to 3 months.

Grab and go. Thaw a muffin overnight in the fridge or microwave for 20–30 seconds. Pair with coffee or tea for a gut-friendly breakfast or snack.

Why These Muffins Work for Gut Health

- **Inulin:** A prebiotic fiber that feeds beneficial gut bacteria, promoting satiety and reducing cravings.

- **Hazelnut flour:** High in fiber and low to moderate amounts of LA to support gut microbiome diversity.
- **Butter:** Contains C15:0 for energy and gut-lining support.
- **Low sugar:** Minimal sweeteners prevent blood sugar spikes, keeping cravings at bay.

———

Mara Bakes Muffins with Her Niece Who Is a Royal Pain

Mara lifted the small package delivered just that morning to her doorstep, surprised at how heavy it was. Once inside, she opened the box and inspected the label on the bottle: "High-Fiber Chicory Inulin."

The supplement was a prebiotic fiber powder that supported beneficial gut bacteria and reduced food cravings. It even bolstered feeling full and satisfied after eating. After her probiotics had paid off with less bloating and zero midnight heartburn this was the next step.

She brought it into the house, just in time for a baking party with her young niece, Kari. The "baking party" was really a favor to her sister who needed a mental health day, but it was a good excuse to try the new prebiotic muffin recipe from Dr. Ellis's cookbook.

"What's that?" Kari scowled and crinkled her little features at the new powder.

"It's an ingredient," Mara said, short. She pulled back her long, dark hair and prepared the table for baking. Kari eyed her from the side and brushed her blond pigtails over her shoulders. "I like sugar. Not this stuff. It's gross."

Mara tied an apron around her waist. "It's not gross. It's healthy."

Kari scowled. "I like muffins the regular way."

Mara's chest tightened. She remembered the breathing technique from her yoga instructor years ago. "These are both healthy and delicious at the same time. They have prebiotics in them, which helps your digestion."

Kari puffed her lips.

Mara measured out all the dry ingredients and placed them into a bowl for Kari to stir.

Kari stirred with her scrawny little arm. "Why does it help your gut?"

Mara measured the wet ingredients. "It helps your gut stay strong, so it doesn't leak garbage everywhere."

"Ew," Kari said.

"I know, right?" Mara coaxed, and poured the wet ingredients into a glass bowl. She explained how prebiotics fuel the gut microbiome. To her shock, Kari listened. Mara placed the muffins into the oven, and they played a game of thumb wars while waiting for them to finish baking.

Bzzz! The timer sounded and Mara pulled the muffins from the oven.

"Smells so good!" Kari squealed.

"That's because they are," Mara said, and dished one out onto Kari's plate.

Kari sunk her teeth into it and screeched with delight. Her little toes curled. "It's the best ever!"

By the time Kari's mom returned, Mara and Kari had bonded over the muffins. And Mara had stocked up on plenty of them to eat throughout the week to support her gut.

CHAPTER 19

Additional Gut Gem–Friendly Supplements

On your journey to better gut health, certain nutritional supplements can help restore balance, improve digestion, support cellular health, and boost immunity. You may already be familiar with some, such as vitamin D, B vitamins, and magnesium. Others, such as C 15:0, may be completely new to you. In this chapter, we will view familiar supplements through the lens of gut health and explore nutrients that support cellular health.

C15:0 Helps Your Cells Heal from PUFS

If you're serious about shaking off the effects of a diet loaded with PUFS, you'll want to prioritize dislodging the linoleic acid that has accumulated in your cells for years. This is where a new-on-the-scene fatty acid—pentadecanoic acid, otherwise known as C15:0—steps into the spotlight.

The harsh truth is that linoleic acid (LA) has a half-life of around 680 days—nearly two full years. Even if you quit PUFS cold turkey right now, you'll still walk around with a backlog of PUFS saturating your tissues for quite some time. Your body just doesn't magically decide to flush everything out the moment you change your diet. For many months—possibly years, depending on how much you put back in on a daily basis—your cells are forced to function in an environment riddled with PUFS, which is prone to peroxidation.

That's the frustration: You're doing everything right by choosing stable saturated fats like butter and coconut oil, and avoiding PUFS-filled foods, yet you might still feel locked into a cycle of mild fatigue, random aches, or seesawing energy.

The good news is you can speed up the LA clearing process by adding in more C15:0, as it competes with LA for integration into your cell membranes. C15:0 is an odd-chain saturated fat found primarily in dairy products that belongs in a category of its own. Because it's stable, C15:0 won't oxidize the moment you turn on a burner (which is why butter is so great for cooking and frying) or the second your cells produce some heat. Most importantly, C15:0 can accelerate the eviction process for PUFS—no more squatting in your cell membranes!

Picture your cell membranes like little patchwork quilts made up of various fats. The more PUFS you have woven in, the higher your susceptibility to oxidative stress. C15:0, in contrast, is saturated and stable. It can handle heat, oxygen, and general metabolic chaos far better. And thanks to its odd-chain structure, C15:0 actively competes with PUFS for space, essentially pushing PUFS out of the driver's seat. If you've spent years piling on the PUFS, you can bring in C15:0 to cut the process of clearing out the LA in your cells from two to six years to a matter of months or weeks, depending on the location.

As you've learned throughout this book, the removal of PUFS from your cells is important to your metabolic destiny. While contributing to inflammation, free radical production, and overall cellular mayhem, PUFS are more insidious in certain tissues, like the liver and skeletal muscle, where the oxygen flux is high and the turnover of fats is rapid. Without a buildup of PUFS, you could count on those tissues to maintain stable blood sugar, burn energy efficiently, and support robust health.

Over time, C15:0's insertion into the double-layered cell membrane rearranges the membrane's composition into one that is less susceptible to free radical damage and more supportive of your cells' normal operations. Your mitochondria (organelles in cells that use nutrients to produce energy) can then work more effectively and efficiently because they're not battling the inflammatory cascade caused by PUFS.

Rethinking Fats for a Lasting Metabolic Edge

Now, you might be thinking, "If C15:0 is so great, why haven't I heard about it sooner?" Simple answer: It's new to the mainstream. C15:0 challenges the conventional wisdom that lumps every type of saturated fat into the "heart attack on a plate" category. It's also not widely available in supplement form, and the forms that do exist are expensive, especially if you're aiming for the 1 to 2 grams a day that many believe is necessary to get meaningful results in displacing PUFS. The daily dose is large compared to the 100 milligrams found in some general "health blends." Sure, 100 milligrams might do something, but if you're trying to uproot a large backlog of PUFS, you'll probably need more.

Current costs are another factor. If you were taking up to 2 grams of C15:0 a day, you could easily spend hundreds of dollars (and depending on the brand, up to $1,000) per month. On the bright side, the market is rapidly evolving. New companies are racing to deliver more affordable forms of C15:0.

If you're considering trying a C15:0 supplement, you should do your homework. Compare products and look for signs of third-party testing and pharmaceutical-grade certifications. Nobody wants to drop serious cash on a supplement that's subpar or doesn't contain what it claims. Also keep in mind that research on high-dose C15:0 in humans is still in the early stages. Most of what we know comes from preclinical studies, with human trials just beginning to emerge.

If you're on a budget, a moderate dose can still be beneficial. You'll displace PUFS at a slower pace, but you'll eventually see improvements if you're also cutting PUFS from your diet. The synergy from limiting the incoming flow of PUFS plus actively pushing out what's lodged in your tissues with C15:0 is far more effective.

C15:0's robust presence in your membranes will also help your insulin receptors, hormones, and neurotransmitter systems function more smoothly. Think about it: If your membranes are stabilized, the proteins embedded in them can do their jobs without grappling with microenvironments that are forever flipping from fluid to rigid, thanks to oxidative hits. Some people, therefore, report enhanced energy, reduced joint aches, and steadier moods once they've started to incorporate C15:0.

You may also wonder how this approach compares to loading up on omega-3 fats, which also help displace some of the harmful fats in your membranes. Omega-3 is great, but it's still unsaturated, meaning it's prone to oxidation. C15:0 is saturated and therefore resistant to the damage that plagues unsaturated fats. That's not to say you should ditch omega-3 altogether. Animal-based omega-3s have essential roles. Nevertheless, C15:0's resilience might give you the upper hand if your body is grappling with high oxidative pressure.

If you decide to give C15:0 a real shot, track how you feel. Notice if your energy levels stay more consistent, if your skin looks better, if you can handle stress a bit more gracefully, and/or if your craving patterns shift. Eventually, as you transition away from high PUFS and stock your membranes with more stable saturated fats like C15:0, you might hit a sweet spot where your energy feels robust and your inflammatory issues recede.

Once you've toppled your old backlog of PUFS and stabilized your cellular membranes, you can reevaluate whether you want to maintain a higher dose of C15:0 or if you're content to let your normal diet be your primary source. No single supplement works like a magic wand, and C15:0 is no exception. But if you're dedicated to fast-tracking the displacement of PUFS and serious about your metabolic future, C15:0 deserves a spot in the conversation.

Other Supplements to Support Gut Healing

Your body needs multiple nutrients for optimal gut health and overall health. To support your gut-health journey, the following supplements are worth considering.

Vitamin D

Vitamin D is vital for immunity and bone health, and it also plays important roles in the gut. It boosts the presence of butyrate-producing bacteria, suppresses inflammation, and helps strengthen the tight junctions between the cells in your gut lining and the mucus layer that protects the lining.

On a more general level, vitamin D is essential for regulating thousands of genes. Optimal vitamin D levels lower the risk of many diseases, including cancer, heart disease, and autoimmune disorders.

The body manufactures vitamin D naturally when your skin is exposed to sunlight. A lack of sun exposure is a main reason people are deficient in vitamin D. Many also work long hours indoors, and slather on sunscreen when they do go outside. If any of those conditions apply to you, particularly if you have been consuming large amounts of PUFS (which make your skin cells more vulnerable to sun damage), you would benefit from supplementation.

When supplementing with vitamin D, you also need magnesium and vitamin K2. These nutrients work synergistically, and imbalances can occur if one is taken in isolation at high doses. The optimal strategy is to take all three together: vitamin D3, magnesium, and vitamin K2. Magnesium also helps your mitochondria produce plenty of ATP, the fuel that your cells need to function.

The average adult with no sun exposure should aim for about 8,000 units of D3, 400 milligrams of magnesium, and 150–200 micrograms of K2 daily. Remember, individual needs may vary. To fine-tune your supplementation, have your vitamin D levels tested twice a year. For optimal health benefits, aim for a level between 60 and 80 ng/mL (150 to 200 nmol/L).

B Complex

B vitamins—especially thiamine (B1) and riboflavin (B2)—help your gut microbes make Gut Gems like butyrate. Gut bacteria also produce thiamine, which supports energy metabolism and nervous system function, and folate (B9), which supports detox, mood, mental health, and the production of red and white blood cells. If your gut bacteria are depleted, you may be running low on these nutrients too.

Because B vitamins work best as a team, it's smart to take a full B complex rather than singling out just one. And when it comes to B9, check your label: you want folate, not folic acid. Folate is the natural form found in foods like fruits, vegetables, legumes, and nuts. Folic acid is the synthetic version used in most supplements and fortified grains. While your body handles whole-food folate just fine, excess folic acid has been linked to unwanted effects.

Polyphenols

Polyphenols are natural antioxidants found in plant foods such as fruits, vegetables, herbs, teas, and spices. They're responsible for the vibrant colors in foods such as berries, red onions, and purple cabbage. These compounds play a vital role in reducing oxidative stress and inflammation and supporting the balance of your gut microbiome.

Other Supplements to Support Gut Healing

Supplement	Gut-Specific Benefits	How to Use
C15:0 (Pentadecanoic acid)	✓ Supports gut barrier integrity ✓ Reduces inflammation ✓ Promotes cellular resilience	100–1,000 mg/day (start low and work up)
Vitamin D3	✓ Strengthens gut lining ✓ Enhances immune regulation ✓ Promotes healthy microbiome balance	2,000–8,000 IU/day with meals; check blood levels (40–60 ng/mL)
Vitamin K2	✓ Works synergistically with D3 ✓ May reduce calcification and support mucosal tissue health	159–200 mcg/day, ideally with Vitamin D3; use MK-7 form for better results
Magnesium	✓ Relieves constipation ✓ Supports gut muscle relaxation ✓ Reduces gut-related anxiety and cramps	200–500 mg/day; use magnesium glycinate or citrate depending on need
B Complex	✓ Supports energy metabolism in gut cells ✓ Reduces stress-related gut symptoms ✓ Supports microbiota diversity	Daily, preferably a methylated B complex with active B12 and folate
Grape-Seed Extract	✓ Polyphenol-rich; promotes beneficial bacteria ✓ Reduces inflammation and oxidative stress	100–300 mg/day with meals
Green Tea Extract (EGCG)	✓ Increases microbiome diversity ✓ Anti-inflammatory and antimicrobial properties	250–500 mg/day; take earlier in the day to avoid sleep disruption from the caffeine
Curcumin (from turmeric)	✓ Supports healing of the gut lining ✓ Potent anti-inflammatory ✓ Helps with IBS/IBD symptoms	500–1,000 mg/day with black pepper (piperine) or liposomal formulation
Quercetin	✓ Reduces gut-related histamine reactions ✓ Supports gut barrier integrity ✓ Eases food sensitivities	250–500 mg/day; cycle 6–8 weeks on, 2 weeks off for best effect

Fig. 24: When trying new supplements, add one at a time and wait one to two weeks before adding another so you can assess the effectiveness of each.

Polyphenols have an impressive list of gut-supportive properties. Acting as prebiotics and fostering the growth of helpful gut microbes that in turn produce Gut Gems, they can reduce pathogenic bacteria, inhibit enzymes that would otherwise digest resistant starch before it reaches the colon, calm systemic inflammation, and strengthen the gut barrier.

Foods rich in polyphenols include green tea, dark chocolate, apples, red onions, turmeric, rosemary, and thyme. If your gut isn't ready for these foods, consider supplementing with:

- Grape-seed extract
- Green tea extract
- Curcumin (from turmeric)
- Quercetin capsules

—————

Mara Creates Cellular Feng Shui

Mara frowned at the new bottle in her kitchen; she swore it was saying, "Riddle me this." It arrived just hours ago that morning in a climate-controlled pouch, wrapped in insulation and stamped with three certification logos she didn't recognize. The label read "C15:0—Odd-Chain Saturated Fat for Metabolic Resilience."

Just days earlier Mara learned about C15:0 during a podcast interview with Dr. Ellis, who made mitochondrial resilience sound like a personal superpower. While Mara didn't buy into every new supplement trending online, she *did* believe in tracking patterns. Her gut had already transformed once—from constant rebellion to quiet cooperation—when she added probiotics and prebiotic inulin. Mara smiled at the bottle and thought, *This new addition might take my health to a new level.*

Mara attempted to decipher her bottle of "C15:0—Odd-Chain Saturated Fat for Metabolic Resilience." She reread part of the instructions she'd noticed the night before: "C15:0 displaces PUFS in your membranes, stabilizes receptors, and helps quiet oxidative stress." She liked the sound of that. "It's like cellular feng shui," she muttered, and rinsed her blender.

After three weeks of "cellular feng shui," she felt something had shifted; subtle changes but they were undeniable. Mara ran longer distances each week. Her post-sprint energy lasted longer.

Mara's running partner, Sarah, noticed something new. "Your skin looks amazing!" she told Mara. "It's so clear and bright. You'll have to give me your dermatologist's contact info."

Mara felt the glow of the compliment and blushed, "No dermatologist. It's all because my gut is healthier now."

><

CHAPTER 20

A Trifecta of Lifestyle Factors to Enhance Gut Health: Stress, Sleep, and Exercise

Your gut community needs more than just fiber, probiotics, prebiotics, and supplements to remain healthy and balanced. Lifestyle factors such as stress, sleep, and exercise can also have an impact on your gut microbiome. Luckily, even small shifts in these three lifestyle pillars can work synergistically to restore bacterial balance and Gut Gem production.

Stress: Master It Before It Masters You

When you're under stress, your body releases cortisol, a hormone that helps you cope short term. When cortisol stays elevated, it can weaken your gut lining. This makes it easier for unwanted microbes or particles to slip through and trigger your immune system, leading to inflammation. That inflammation can keep the stress response going. Think of your gut lining like a zipper held closed by proteins called tight junctions. When cortisol remains high, those proteins loosen—like zipper teeth coming apart—allowing substances to leak through. Fortunately, small releases of stress can significantly reduce high cortisol levels.

Here's an easy exercise you can try: Breathe in for four counts, hold for four, exhale for six. Repeat four times. The brief breath hold sends a message to your vagus nerve—your gut-brain hotline—saying that danger has passed.

Other stress-busting techniques include tai chi, yoga, meditation, mindfulness training, psychotherapy, music therapy, and progressive muscle relaxation. When you adopt conscious stress release as a regular habit, over time, your inevitable cortisol spikes won't rise as high or last as long, and the zipper of your gut lining will remain closed.

Sleep: Your Nightly Microbiome Makeover

Experts recommend seven to nine hours of shut-eye for many reasons. One benefit of adequate sleep is gut restoration and repair. During deep sleep, melatonin rises, which tightens the gut lining and spurs friendly bacteria to crank out Gut Gems. When you skip sleep, Gut Gem production diminishes.

To help yourself fall and stay asleep, dim the overhead lights two hours before bed. Bright LEDs fool the brain into thinking it's still daytime. Swap late-night social media scrolling for a warm shower or bath and write down tomorrow's to-do list before you brush your teeth so that you don't have to think about those tasks while you're trying to drift off. Do what you can to remove nagging thoughts from your head before bed to spare yourself middle-of-the-night brain chatter.

One of the most overlooked ways to improve sleep is by getting sunlight in the morning and again around midday. Natural light exposure helps regulate your circadian rhythm by signaling to your brain when it's time to be alert and when to wind down. Without enough bright light during the day—especially in the morning—your body may struggle to produce melatonin at night.

Exercise: Move It to Improve It

Exercise doesn't just benefit your heart and muscles. It also reshapes your gut. Physical activity has been shown to increase the diversity of your gut microbiome and support the growth of beneficial bacteria that produce Gut Gems, including butyrate, acetate, and propionate.

Studies show that regular exercise—especially aerobic or resistance training—can boost levels of Gut Gem–producing bacteria such as *Faecalibacterium prausnitzii*, *Roseburia*, and *Lachnospiraceae* while also increasing overall microbial diversity and mucosal health. Well-trained individuals, including athletes, also tend to have more

Akkermansia muciniphila, a species associated with reduced intestinal inflammation and healthier mucus layers.

This microbiome shift appears to be one way exercise supports cognitive and metabolic health. During exercise, muscle contractions release compounds called myokines, which help protect the brain and enhance gut-microbiome crosstalk. A myokine called irisin, in particular, has been shown to protect the gut lining and may help reverse dysbiosis in conditions such as ulcerative colitis.

So, instead of viewing exercise as a way to burn off dessert, think of it as nourishment for your microbiome. Even moderate activity, such as a brisk twenty-minute walk, can stimulate blood flow to your gut, support microbial diversity, and promote Gut Gem production. Over time, this can help reduce inflammation not just in your gut but throughout your entire body.

If you don't have much free time, try micro-workouts. For example, during TV commercials, knock out ten body-weight squats or a wall sit. These short movement breaks add up. For variety, you can alternate between body-weight resistance and the neighborhood hills.

Putting It All Together: The Lifestyle Audit and Bingo Challenge

First, let's see how well you're taking care of the three vital areas of health with a lifestyle audit. Take out your notebook and draw six columns. Label them as follows: Stress Good, Stress Bad, Sleep Good, Sleep Bad, Move Good, and Move Bad.

Under each "Bad" column, list what went wrong. For example, maybe you blew past lunch, scrolled news on your tablet at midnight, or skipped the stairs. Under each "Good" column, make a note of what went well. Perhaps you tried a breathing exercise or did a few squats while the coffee brewed. Use your audit to plan what you'll do better the next day and write it down on tomorrow's to-do list.

Next, for some fun, cue Gut-Health Bingo! Use the included chart as inspiration for doing little things that support your new gut-healthy lifestyle. Every time you accomplish something listed here, mark it with an X. When you get five in a row, reward yourself with a gut-friendly treat, such as coconut-oil chocolate bark (melt coconut oil, stir in cocoa, possibly some cinnamon, and chill). To make the most of your bingo card, text a picture of it to a friend at the end of each day. Accountability will help you cross off more squares.

Gut-Health Bingo

⭐ B	⭐ I	⭐ N	⭐ G	⭐ O
Lights out by 10:00 p.m.	10-minute stretch	2-minute box-breathing	Walk barefoot on grass	No screens 1 hour before bed
Lunch in sunlight	Dance to one song	Gratitude journaling (3 things)	Power down phone at 9:00 p.m.	Post-meal stroll (10+ mins)
Deep breathing before meals	Yoga or tai chi session	FREE SPACE	Wake up with natural light	Nature break (trees, sky, etc.)
Set a daily movement goal	Legs up the wall (5 mins)	Declutter one small space	Hydrate first thing in morning	Meditate for 5+ minutes
No caffeine after 2:00 p.m.	Phone-free lunch	Write down tomorrow's to-do list before bed	Journal before bed	Take stairs instead of elevator

Fig. 25: Cross off each mini-moment of self-care you complete. When you get five in a row, give yourself a little reward.

—◄

Mara's Inside-Out Makeover

That morning at the gym in downtown Chicago, Mara received compliment after compliment about her skin—comments like "You're glowing" and "You look radiant." She had never given much thought to her skin before, but after all the compliments, Mara felt inspired to reconsider her self-care regimen. Previously she thought there was nothing to be done about the way she looked, really. But her new gut health enhanced her skin entirely. Perhaps she imagined it, but even her eyes were clearer and brighter now.

She could use more of this glow-up in her life. She decided to implement a threefold beauty manifesto: enough sleep, healthy foods, and the right exercise.

That evening, Mara scrolled through videos of "10-minute workouts" on her phone until midnight. *Oops!* By the time she flopped onto her pillow, she felt wired and annoyed. She promised herself to be in bed by 10:00 p.m. from that moment on, and she finally fell asleep.

The following night, Mara dimmed every LED light two hours before bedtime. She brain-dumped the next day's to-do list so she wouldn't think about it, then turned off her laptop and set her phone to airplane mode.

Mara also tracked her stress and exercise. She had to add two habits to her most recent tracking chart. Under stress she wrote "Bad."

Under meals she wrote "Skipped lunch prepping."

Under sleep she noted "Forgot to set phone to airplane mode and notifications woke me up. And I watched random videos for two hours in the middle of the night."

Mara deflated. She was not doing as well as she had hoped. To make things worse, she felt cranky from interrupted sleep. She picked one thing to improve the next day. On a sticky note she wrote "Set phone to airplane mode." She stuck the note to her bathroom mirror, where she would see it before going to bed.

><

CHAPTER 21

Assessing Your Gut Health

An important part of any gut-health restoration plan is a simple assessment of your current status. Assess your gut by noticing when your digestion, mood, and energy levels stray from normal. If you haven't been tracking your sensations, now is the perfect time to start. If you have, it's time to consider getting some basic blood tests done. The reason is to determine if you've been quietly battling metabolic headwinds from too many PUFS. A little reconnaissance goes a long way, especially if you've spent years fighting a mystery war inside your belly.

Your gut is unique. You may have one friend who deals with constipation and another who struggles with diarrhea. You might not have either problem but suffer with bloating, fatigue, mood dips after meals, or waking up exhausted after a solid night's sleep. All are clues that something is off in your gut.

Bloating is often the first red flag, indicating that unfriendly bacteria are producing large amounts of gas. Fatigue that seems to come out of nowhere can be the result of inflamed colonocytes and microbial imbalances that lead to sluggish energy production.

The everyday annoyances that are easy to brush aside can offer real insights into the condition of your colonocytes and microbial crew. There's no reason to live in discomfort or simply not feel your best. With a little patience, you can figure out what your body needs and develop a strategy that addresses the root cause of your symptoms.

Gut-Health-Symptom Checklist

Use the following checklist to assess your symptoms at baseline and again weekly or monthly. Score each symptom on a scale of 0 to 3:

0 = Not at all

1 = Mild (occasional or slight impact)

2 = Moderate (frequent or noticeable impact)

3 = Severe (daily or major impact on life)

Symptom	Score (0–3)
Bloating	
Gas (excessive or foul-smelling)	
Diarrhea	
Constipation	
Abdominal cramping or pain	
Nausea	
Acid reflux or heartburn	
Food cravings (especially sugar)	
Food intolerances or sensitivities	
Brain fog or difficulty focusing	
Fatigue or low energy	
Joint pain or stiffness	
Headaches or migraines	
Skin issues (acne, eczema, rashes)	
Mood swings or irritability	
Anxiety or nervousness	
Depressive symptoms	
Frequent colds or infections	
Sleep disturbances	
Bad breath	

Total Score: _____

You can add your score to your wellness journal and repeat the checklist regularly to track changes. A declining total over time is an indication of improvements in gut health.

Microbiome Tests Are Just One Piece of the Puzzle

At-home microbiome tests offer a glimpse into your gut's microbial balance, revealing if beneficial bacteria are overshadowed by pathogens. However, they're not definitive diagnostic tools. The tests provide a snapshot, influenced by factors such as stress, sleep, and diet. Results focus mainly on identifying harmful bacteria rather than nurturing beneficial strains, often missing newly discovered microbes.

Historically, medicine has prioritized eliminating pathogens over supporting gut repair, so tests rarely highlight the need for beneficial bacteria. Results might show low levels of Gut Gem–producing strains or overgrowth of bacteria that thrive on processed foods. Such news can help you decide whether to increase fiber or focus on healing colonocytes. Treat results as one data point, not a complete guide. Pay attention to how you feel. Calmer digestion, steady energy, and a balanced immune system are your true indicators of progress. Use test insights as motivation, not strict instructions.

At-Home Lab Tests: A Convenient Way to Fine-Tune Your Gut and Metabolism

Another big factor in your metabolic journey is insulin resistance. The more PUFS you've piled on, the higher the risk that your cells aren't using glucose well. If you suspect your metabolism is on the rocks, checking your insulin sensitivity by calculating your Homeostatic Model Assessment for Insulin Resistance (HOMA-IR) might be the wake-up call you need. This simple blood test tells you how resistant your cells are to insulin, and you can purchase it for under twenty-five dollars from online labs without a doctor's order. Affordable access to the kits allows you to take the test repeatedly and track your progress over time. Rather than guess, you can objectively measure how your insulin sensitivity improves as you ease off PUFS and shore up your gut lining.

Direct-to-consumer lab tests are designed for you to do right at home. You don't have to make an appointment with a physician to obtain a prescription. If you need to fast beforehand, the ability to do it at home, according to your own schedule, is a big plus. Many companies can mail you a dried blood spot kit that merely requires you to prick your finger, dab a few drops of blood on a little card, and send it back. You'll typically get your results in about a week. Companies offering these kits have streamlined the process to get your results into your hands fast, often with a user-friendly interface so you can make sense of the numbers.

If you're trying to keep tabs on something like insulin resistance—or any gut-related marker—the home-test approach is a game changer. For one option, check out the Mercola Health Coach app. We offer at-home lab tests at some of the lowest prices around.

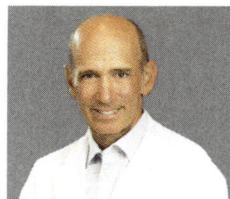

Scan this QR code to get FREE access to the Mercola Health Coach app. This tool allows you to log your meals, track your macronutrient ratios, and monitor your progress over time.

At Mercola, we take it a step further by combining your test results with detailed health questionnaires to deliver a personalized report that goes beyond the numbers. Think of it as the insight you'd get from an in-depth consultation—without the specialist price tag. Our system uses advanced, real-time analysis to scan your health history and uncover meaningful patterns, saving you time and money while giving you actionable answers.

In truth, you will end up with a broader, more up-to-date analysis than any single brief appointment could provide. Instead of having one experienced physician to deliver a quick assessment, you gain answers from a system that combs through massive amounts of research to link your health history with your lab results and pinpoint exactly what's relevant to you.

The detailed, personalized feedback we tack on is free. You pay no consult charges beyond the cost of the test. Also, once you submit your information, you become part of one of the largest clinical trials on record. As we guide you, the real-world feedback we gather will help refine and improve our innovative protocols.

This level of insight simply hasn't been on the table before for those who want genuine clarity about what's happening with their gut health. And you get all this without slugging through the usual red tape. All the while, you can contribute to groundbreaking research that keeps pushing health recommendations forward.

HOMA-IR: Your Metabolic Crystal Ball

Insulin resistance is closely tied to gut health and cellular function. Diets high in PUFS disrupt your cell membranes and impair how your cells respond to insulin. Over time, this makes it harder for glucose to enter your cells efficiently, prompting your body to release even more insulin. The result is a cycle of rising insulin levels, chronic inflammation, and increasing metabolic stress that eventually leads to insulin resistance followed by full-blown diabetes.

HOMA-IR is an inexpensive test that uses your insulin and fasting glucose levels to give you a snapshot of how well you handle carbs. The formula for determining HOMA-IR is to multiply your fasting insulin (measured in uIU/mL) by your fasting glucose (measured in mg/mL) and divide by 405.

Here's the breakdown of possible results:

- Less than 1.0: insulin sensitive (which is what you want)
- Between 1.1 and 2.9: early insulin resistance
- Above 2.9: significant insulin resistance

For example, if your fasting insulin were 10 uIU/mL, and your fasting glucose were 100 mg/mL, you'd multiply the two to get 1,000. Next, you would divide 1,000 by 405. Rounding up, you would get 2.5, indicating early insulin resistance.

If your HOMA-IR score is above 1.1, you need to cut PUFS and work to improve your gut microbiome. At present, the gold standard in measuring insulin resistance is the euglycemic hyperinsulinemic clamp. Unfortunately, this test is only used in research settings due to the time and cost involved. The process requires spending a whole day in a research lab, hooked up to IV lines of insulin and glucose, while a team monitors and tweaks the rates to keep your blood sugar steady. While extremely accurate, this is not a test that you can get at your local clinic. Even if it were somehow commercially available, this method would easily cost over $1,000.

That's what makes HOMA-IR so appealing. It's relatively inexpensive and can be ordered online without a prescription. If you track your HOMA-IR every couple of months, you'll know if your diet adjustments—like removing seed oils and eating stable fats—are making a difference in your metabolic picture. Nothing is more encouraging than watching your insulin levels inch back toward normal.

Lab Results Unlocked

If your HOMA-IR test shows your fasting glucose is creeping up, don't panic. It's valuable information you can use for motivation to take action. Start by cutting more PUFS and, if needed, support your gut with an *Akkermansia* postbiotic or probiotic (depending on the current state of your gut), or C15:0 supplement until you're ready to reintroduce more fiber. Take the reins now and plan to recheck your labs in two or three months.

Some people like to track their progress visually. You could circle your first lab result in bold red on a whiteboard or notebook, then write down your follow-up number a few weeks later. Watching that number drop can feel like a high-five for every PUFS-filled snack you skipped. Even better, when real food starts to truly satisfy you, your metabolic health gets a serious upgrade.

Just remember—lab tests are tools, not verdicts. If your numbers don't shift as quickly as you hoped, don't dismiss the wins you *can* feel. More stable energy, smoother digestion, and fewer cravings are all signs you're heading in the right direction.

Above all, having clear data gives you a major advantage. It tells you what's working and what might need tweaking—so you're not left guessing.

Tools for Measuring PUFS and Other Markers

Another useful blood test is the red blood cell (RBC) fatty acid profile, which directly measures how your dietary fat choices are influencing your cell structure—especially the reduction of linoleic acid (LA). It does this by detecting early changes in the fats that make up your red blood cell membranes.

Red blood cells live for about 115 to 120 days, but shifts in LA levels can begin to show in as little as four weeks. Home testing kits, like the OmegaQuant Complete ($90–$110), offer a simple finger-stick option and provide detailed results, including your individual LA percentage and your total omega-3 index. If your LA drops below 8 percent and your omega-3 index rises above 8 percent, it's a strong sign that healthier fats are displacing the more inflammatory ones—clear evidence that your dietary changes are reshaping your cell membranes. Pairing a fasting insulin or HOMA-IR test with the RBC fatty acid profile gives you a dual view: the metabolic effects of your fat reset and the structural shifts happening at the cellular level.

For a more budget-friendly option, you can substitute the fatty acid test with a high-sensitivity CRP (hs-CRP) test, which serves as a marker of inflammation. It often drops within weeks of cutting out seed oils. The Quest Diagnostics cash price is typically around fifty dollars. While hs-CRP can't confirm that LA is being replaced by more stable fats, it offers an early signal that overall inflammation is on the decline. Keep in mind, though, that hs-CRP can spike during acute infections such as colds or the flu, so if you've been sick recently, wait a couple of weeks before retesting to get a more accurate picture.

While tests aren't mandatory to heal your gut, they can speed up your learning curve, especially if you are data driven. Instead of guessing which adjustments are moving the needle, you'll see the chemical story unfold in real time. However, don't worry if the costs will strain your budget. An old-fashioned daily journal—plus an occasional HOMA-IR for good measure—might be all you need to stay on track.

Gut-Health Stages: From Damage to Healing

The following table can help you discern how the steps you're taking to improve your gut health are making a difference. Use it in conjunction with the Gut-Health-Symptom Checklist provided previously in this chapter to track your overall progress.

Gut-Health Stages: From Damage to Healing

	Damaged Gut	Healing Gut
Digestion	Frequent bloating, gas, constipation, diarrhea, or cramping	More regular bowel movements, less bloating, improved tolerance to foods
Cravings	Strong cravings for sugar, carbs, caffeine, or salty snacks	Reduced cravings, balanced appetite, increased satisfaction after meals
Energy Levels	Fatigue, especially after meals; energy crashes	More sustained energy, fewer slumps during the day
Cognitive Function	Brain fog, forgetfulness, difficulty focusing	Sharper thinking, improved memory and concentration
Mood	Irritability, anxiety, mood swings, depressive episodes	More emotional stability, calmness, and resilience
Skin	Breakouts, rashes, eczema, dull complexion	Clearer, more vibrant skin; reduction in inflammation
Immunity	Frequent colds, infections; slow wound healing	Fewer illnesses, quicker recovery time, improved overall immunity
Pain and Inflammation	Joint aches, stiffness, chronic inflammation	Reduced pain, improved mobility, less stiffness
Sleep	Trouble falling asleep or staying asleep, waking tired	Deeper, more restful sleep, easier time falling and staying asleep
Reactions to Food	Food sensitivities, bloating or discomfort after eating	Better tolerance to a wider range of foods, less digestive upset
Weight	Unexplained gain or difficulty losing weight, bloating	Stabilized or more manageable weight, reduced bloating
Overall Well-Being	Feeling unwell without clear reason, general discomfort	Feeling more balanced, comfortable, and confident in your body

Fig. 26: Prioritizing your gut health pays off in a large variety of ways that extend well past improved digestion.

Remember:

- Healing is nonlinear. It's normal to have flare-ups during the process.
- Celebrate small wins, such as more regular digestion and clearer thinking.

Finding the Starting Point for True Healing

So, how do you pull all of this together into a cohesive plan? Step 1 is paying attention to your day-to-day gut signals. They include which meals cause trouble, how much bloat you're living with, and whether your bowel habits are stable or all over the place. Step 2 is deciding if you want to gather additional data: a microbiome check, a HOMA-IR reading, or a look at how much PUFS might be flowing through your bloodstream.

The goal is to figure out whether your gut is ready for bigger dietary changes such as reintroducing fiber or exploring supplements. If you force change before you're ready, you might sabotage some of the progress you've already made. By checking in with yourself (and, if needed, your labs), you'll know when it's time to embrace new foods, and start adding in postbiotic, prebiotic or probiotic supplements, or eat more fiber.

Set Yourself Up for Success

If there's one takeaway from all this, it's that you deserve to know what's happening in your gut. You want to know how your colonocytes are holding up, whether your beneficial microbes are in need of backup, and if your insulin levels are in need of attention. That might mean a self-guided approach with a gut journal, or it could involve specific lab tests to shine a light on hidden metabolic traps. It's your call.

The specifics can vary, but the concept is universal: When you get real about your starting point, you're far more likely to arrive at the destination you desire. Ultimately the best recipe for success is targeted actions based on actual intel rather than leaps of faith.

><

Mara's Stress at the Zoo Offices Ruins Everything

Mara sipped her morning coffee wearily at her desk in the Chicago Zoo offices, and she scowled at the stacks of papers and reports piled on her desk. As a program manager for the Chicago Zoo,

Mara had many responsibilities, including monitoring data on the animals. Engrossed in her work, she was distracted by multiple messages pinging her inbox:

ORANGUTANS: HELP NEEDED ASAP

Several males had fought over a new female. *Predictable,* Mara thought as she rolled her eyes. But apparently the fight was quite bad, and one of the orangutans sustained a severe concussion. The zookeeper rang the emergency vets. The alert put everyone in the zoo offices on edge. Although Mara was not responsible for handling the orangutans directly, she held all the data on them, and the emergency responders' stress was contagious.

The emergency vets filed in, in red uniforms, carrying cases and backpacks filled with medical equipment.

Mara and the groundskeeper fidgeted by the glass enclosure. The wounded orangutan wailed in pain.

An emergency vet with a downturned mustache turned to Mara, "Does he have any allergies?"

"What?" Mara said stupidly. Her gut dipped through the cement floor.

"Allergies," he pressed. "I need to administer treatment but the ape could die if I give him the wrong thing. You have to tell me now."

Mara heard the words "die" and "now" and her knees went weak. Cortisol pumped through her neck. Stress gripped her gut in a tight knot. "I'll just . . . pull that up . . . in a file . . . somewhere . . ." she muttered, nauseous.

"No!" the vet cried. "We need to know now! We have to save his life!"

It sounded as though everything were underwater. Mara could not feel her face. She could look in her files but she wasn't that organized, really. She had no idea about orangutans. She was still getting used to her new role at the zoo. The stress made her gut dip. Her head went dizzy and faint.

Mara shook her head, "No allergies," she said in almost a whisper. Although she had no idea, and it was practically a lie.

The vets poured into the glass enclosure and scrambled into place around the orangutan. They administered a shot to him, but his mouth foamed in an allergic reaction, and Mara could hardly look. She snapped her head away and ran into the offices.

That night, unable to sleep, Mara massaged the tension in her neck. Her gut bloated and twisted into a knot.

I had no idea stress impacted my gut so much, she thought. Mara rolled out of bed and wandered to the kitchen. She found a block of cheese and carved a hunk of it with a knife. She nibbled at the cheddar. If only she knew exactly what was in her gut, really.

Mara paused. She could figure it out; she could take a microbiome test. She flipped open her laptop and discovered she could order an at-home microbiome test. The fact that she wouldn't have to leave work this week for a doctor's appointment was a godsend.

I am just as important as those orangutans. She chewed her cheese angrily. *Every aspect of their health is tested every month. I'm going to test mine, too!*

HOMA-IR testing could confirm whether lingering issues—amplified by stress—were still sabotaging her gut. As someone who loved data, even tracking how many pounds she deadlifted from lift to lift, Mara had always appreciated concrete numbers. Lab statistics could offer the necessary structure and clarity. She would be thorough with her health data.

If only she could have done the same for the orangutans.

CHAPTER 22

Building Your Gut-Healing Plan

Healing a damaged gut is not a quick fix, despite the allure of instant solutions. Cutting out problematic foods or taking one-off probiotics over a short period often yields minimal results. A structured, phased plan that recognizes the gut's complexity and sensitivity is key.

After years of processed foods, weakened colonocytes, and imbalanced microbes, superficial fixes rarely work. An effective approach incorporates progressive steps that are adjusted to your unique body and lifestyle. While you've already been given—and perhaps experimented with—all of these steps already, here's a quick recap. This plan now follows a repair to reseed sequence centered on *Akkermansia*: Phase 1 uses postbiotic *Akkermansia* (Amuc_1100 signal) to tighten the barrier; Phase 2 introduces live *Akkermansia* with gentle prebiotics to restore robust Gut Gem production.

Step 1: Say Goodbye to PUFS

When PUFS are allowed to disrupt your gut microbiome, they undermine healing efforts. The small amounts of PUFS that naturally occur in foods such as nuts and seeds are not the problem. Eliminating the highly refined industrial seed oils that are responsible for destabilizing your gut, however, is a lifelong habit for lasting gut health.

Step 2: Repair the Gut Lining with Postbiotic *Akkermansia*

Postbiotics—also known as metabiotics, biogenics, or simply metabolites—are bioactive compounds produced by bacteria as a result of their metabolism or after they die and break apart.

When fiber "backfires," start with a *postbiotic* form of *Akkermansia*—pasteurized cells or their outer-membrane vesicles—that naturally carry the repair cue Amuc_1100. As mentioned previously, this protein helps tighten junctions and support epithelial renewal without feeding a dysbiotic blaze. Just remember, enteric coating or microencapsulation is strongly preferred so that Amuc_1100 will be able to bypass stomach acid and bile; unprotected ("naked") protein typically loses most of its activity before reaching the colon. Stay in this phase for several weeks to a few months while keeping meals low in PUFS and managing stress.

Step 3: Reseed with Live *Akkermansia* and Gentle Prebiotics

Once the gut lining shows signs of repair—such as more regular stools, less bloat and fewer food reactions—start adding live *Akkermansia,* overlapping with the postbiotic for two to four weeks, along with small amounts of well-tolerated prebiotic foods to feed gut bacteria without reigniting bloat. Examples: a tablespoon of cooked-and-cooled rice or potato, or a small shake-in of green-banana flour in yogurt. Increase the amount of prebiotic foods every 1–2 weeks if comfort holds. If gas or urgency returns, pause the introduction of new prebiotics for three to five days (but continue the postbiotic and live *Akkermansia),* then start adding in new prebiotic foods again at half the prior amount. This reseed step restores the oxygen-poor ecosystem that drives your own production of butyrate, propionate, and acetate—your indispensable Gut Gems.

Step 4: Experiment with Adding More Fiber

Once your gut is stable—digestion is smooth, bloating is rare, and bowel movements are consistent—you can cautiously reintroduce fiber. Fiber feeds the beneficial bacteria you've reestablished by taking live *Akkermansia* with gentle prebiotics, but jumping in too soon risks setbacks such as gas, cramps, and immune flare-ups if your gut is still fragile.

Start small with a tablespoon or two daily from well-cooked vegetables, fruit, prebiotics (for example, onions, bananas, oats), or resistant starch (for example, cooked and cooled potatoes or cooked and cooled rice). Increase by a tablespoon or two weekly, monitoring for digestive distress and pausing if needed.

When fiber is tolerated, it signals deep healing: robust colonocytes (from Amuc_1100-guided repair) and a diverse microbial community (from reseeding with live *Akkermansia*). Fiber then enhances this balance, fueling Gut Gem production for effortless digestion and a thriving gut.

Step 5: Add in Exercise

As we covered previously, regular physical activity benefits gut health in multiple ways: It supports regular digestion, reduces inflammation, boosts stress resilience, helps stabilize blood sugar and insulin levels, and fosters microbiome diversity. It's a wonder drug for whole-body health, but the gut particularly benefits. You can start small with a daily walk and gentle stretching and work your way up to 150–300 minutes (2½–5 hours) of moderate-intensity exercise per week.

Ideally include a mix of exercises, including resistance training, to cover all the bases. Just remember, you don't need to push yourself to the limit. Listen to your body. Movement should energize and balance you, not exhaust or inflame you.

><

Mara Crafts a Plan for Sarah and Others

One morning, in her kitchen, Mara drew a picture of a road and felt a bit whimsical about it. Sarah had asked for a road map for her own gut-health journey, but she probably wasn't expecting an actual map with a road. Ha! Mara felt quite clever. She set down her pens and detailed the various steps for Sarah: Remove PUFS; add stable fats; introduce *Akkermansia* and other probiotics; and finally add fiber.

Mara made a special note of it on the side of the map. Only when digestion felt smooth should she reintroduce fiber. Soft veggies first. Then maybe cooled potatoes. A tablespoon at a time.

She also added that exercise was a gut-healthy move, and Sarah certainly had that covered. Lastly, sleep quality. Mara drew a little icon on the map of someone fast asleep.

Later that day, at the gym, Mara handed Sarah the visual road-map drawing.

"This is for me?" Sarah beamed. "I love it!"

"You can put it on your fridge. It'll remind you."

The two women hugged, and Mara felt as though her journey had come full circle. She had even helped someone else.

><

CHAPTER 23

Low-Toxin Cooking:
A Delicious Start

Cooking at home gives you control—over ingredients, oils, additives, and ultimately your gut. When every bite either supports or sabotages your healing, this control becomes your superpower. Yes, cooking takes effort—but it doesn't have to be complicated. A few foundational strategies can transform your meals from inflammatory landmines to gut-soothing medicine. Whether you batch-prep on Sunday or toss together a five-minute stir-fry, your kitchen can be your most powerful healing tool.

Step 1: Stock Gut-Smart Staples

Skip the stress of last-minute takeout by keeping your fridge and freezer stocked with whole-food essentials:

- Frozen meats and veggies (check labels for clean sourcing)
- Precooked rice or potatoes (chilled for resistant starch)
- Ready-to-eat probiotic condiments like sauerkraut or pickles—but only if they're naturally fermented. Look for pickles made in a salt-water brine (not vinegar) and labeled as "fermented" or "naturally fermented." Ingredients should list water, salt, and spices—not vinegar—as the base. They're usually refrigerated and may mention "live cultures" or "probiotic" on the label. Shelf-stable, vinegar-based, or pasteurized pickles do not contain probiotics.
- Stable cooking fats like butter, ghee, tallow, or coconut oil

Just having these on hand means you can throw together a fast meal—like browned ground beef with frozen spinach and reheated rice—without sacrificing your gut goals.

If you're craving a crunch, make your own real-food snacks instead of reaching for packaged chips. Thinly slice zucchini, eggplant, or sweet potato and lightly brush with coconut oil or ghee. Sprinkle with salt and any gut-friendly spices you love (such as turmeric or rosemary) and bake at a low temperature (around 250°F or 121°C) until crisp.

They won't taste like ultra-processed chips, but they'll satisfy your crunch craving without the PUFS overload. Over time, your taste buds will adapt and real food will start tasting better than the ultra-processed stuff you thought you couldn't live without. And your gut will thank you—quietly, reliably, meal after meal.

Step 2: Upgrade the Oils, Upgrade the Outcome

Industrial seed oils such as soybean or canola are silent saboteurs. Swap them for gut-stabilizing fats that can withstand heat without oxidizing. Use:

- Butter or ghee for sautéing
- Tallow for high-heat searing
- Coconut oil or butter for baking or crisping vegetables

These stable fats not only protect your microbiome. They also support butyrate production—fuel for your gut lining.

Step 3: Layer in Gut-Healing Ingredients

Once your meals are PUFS free, build in foods that actively support your microbiome:

- Resistant starch from cooled rice, oats, or potatoes
- Fermented foods such as kefir, kimchi, or sauerkraut
- Fiber-rich foods such as cooked carrots, zucchini, oats, bananas, or apples
- Spices such as turmeric, cumin, and oregano for flavor and anti-inflammatory benefits

Don't overdo it—especially with ferments and fiber. Start with a spoonful and scale up only if your digestion responds well.

Step 4: Meal Prep with Purpose

Even one hour of prep can change your week. Roast veggies, steam gentle greens, brown meat, and cook starches in bulk. Cool and store them for grab-and-go meals or fast reheats.

- Reheat starches to increase resistant starch.
- Add broth to sautéed meals for moisture and minerals.
- Top bowls with fermented condiments for a microbial boost.
- Use apple cider vinegar, ginger, garlic, or lemon juice in marinades to support digestion.

Kitchen Confidence Tips

You don't have to be a master chef to make gut-friendly cooking part of your routine. The first step is to give yourself permission to experiment. In fact, get ready to make a few flops along the way. You might overcook something the first time or decide the flavor combo you chose was terrible. That's okay. Every attempt teaches you what your taste buds and your belly respond to.

You may want to pick one or two basic cooking methods that you feel comfortable using. That might be pan-searing meats or roasting them in the oven. In time, gradually expand your repertoire. If you can roast a chicken in butter, you can do the same with a pork loin or a piece of fish. If you can sauté onions in tallow, you can sauté peppers and mushrooms.

Once you get the hang of the method, you can get creative with spices or marinades. A pinch of sea salt, a grind of pepper, or a dash of herbs can turn an otherwise bland dish into a new favorite. Experiment with whatever makes your kitchen smell delicious.

Simple Meal Plan Ideas

When you're exhausted or short on time, you need recipes that require zero brainpower. Here's a flexible formula: Choose a protein you tolerate—like ground beef, chicken thighs, or salmon. Season with salt and optional herbs, then cook it in your stable fat of choice.

Pair it with a soft, gut-friendly starch such as cooked white rice, mashed potatoes, or oven-roasted sweet potatoes. If your digestion allows, add a gentle veggie such as peeled zucchini, carrots, or spinach. Still in a delicate phase? Skip the veggies but include a small portion of white rice. Even this basic combo is far better than grabbing takeout loaded with seed oils and additives. You'll feel fuller, calmer, and more in control—without needing a fancy recipe or plan.

A crowd-favorite approach is the "one-pan wonder." Toss a few pieces of chicken in a baking dish, add a bit of melted butter, sprinkle with herbs, and bake. If you're at the stage where you can handle certain veggies, throw them in the pan, too. Sweet potatoes (in small cubes) can soak up the butter and turn into a caramelized delight. An alternative is a handful of chopped carrots. Let the oven do the hard work while you catch up on your day. When the timer dings, you'll have a hearty, gut-friendly meal.

For a quick lunch or a swift dinner, ground beef can be your best friend. Brown the meat on a stovetop, drain any excess liquid, and toss in seasonings that don't irritate your gut. You could add a spoonful of plain tomato sauce if you're tolerant. Just let it simmer into the meat. Pour the cooked mixture over a bed of something neutral that you can handle, such as a small portion of pureed root vegetables or white rice. Suddenly you have a dish that's reminiscent of a comfort-food classic.

Gut-Friendly Recipe Challenge

Each week, pick one new gut-friendly recipe to try. Maybe you spotted an idea online or heard a friend rave about a dish that relies on butter instead of seed oils. Challenge yourself to whip it up, even if it's a bit outside your culinary comfort zone.

Keep track of how your creation turns out. Did your belly throw a fit? Was it surprisingly calm afterward? Your log can double as a personal recipe list and a gut-status monitor. Over time, you'll see which meals are "safe bets" for calmer digestion and which ones need some tweaking.

Sharing your results with a supportive friend or online group can make your food adventure more fun. You might trade tips, swap ideas for flavor variations, or bond over the occasional flop. Accountability keeps you motivated to experiment.

Making Toxin-Free Cooking Painless

If you feel overwhelmed by the idea of removing hidden toxins from your kitchen, take a breath. The process can be incremental. Start by clearing out the obvious culprits—bottles of canola, corn, and soybean oil. Replace them with butter, coconut oil, tallow, and ghee. Next, survey your pantry for packaged foods that might be swimming in PUFS or stuffed with odd additives. Gradually swap them out for better alternatives. The point is progress over time, not perfection overnight.

And yes, reading labels might feel tedious at first, but you'll get the hang of it quickly. Over time, you'll have your go-to brands and staples that align with your gut's needs. You might find independent farmers who sell high-quality meats and produce. In addition to being tastier, options by local growers are often free of questionable chemicals that stress your system.

When you realize that a fresh cut of meat or a crisp vegetable can taste fantastic with just a dash of salt and a dab of butter, you might wonder why you ever relied on jarred sauces and marinades.

One underrated trick is to keep a few homemade "foundations" ready. That might be bone broth simmered gently with minimal spices or a batch of shredded slow-cooked beef. Your base then becomes the start for multiple meals: soup one day, stir-fry the next, or a casserole if your belly can handle some veggies. With a little forethought, you can avoid dinnertime panic with handy building blocks that suit your gut-friendly menus.

As you clean up your ingredients, don't forget your cookware—cast iron and stainless steel are solid options that help you avoid PFAS, the hormone-disrupting "forever chemicals" found in most nonstick cookware.

Recipe Customizer: Make It Your Own

One size rarely fits all in the kitchen when managing gut sensitivities. That's why adjusting recipes to suit your personal needs is a must. A certain spice blend might work for you, but your neighbor can't tolerate it. You may need to limit beans, while your coworker can pile them on. The best approach is to see recipes as blueprints, not commandments.

If you are unsure about a dish, consider how you could substitute questionable ingredients for safer alternatives. Could you swap one vegetable for another or omit it altogether without wrecking the meal? Could you reduce the seasoning intensity if you're unsure how your gut will react? Keep notes of your modifications so you remember what worked and what flopped.

Feel free to get creative. If you like the idea of a certain dish but want to jazz up the flavor, experiment with different herbs or moderate amounts of other safe condiments. You might discover a love for turmeric or find that smoked paprika gives a barbecue vibe without the store-bought sauce.

Healing Really Does Start in Your Kitchen

Behind every stable, resilient gut is a series of daily food choices that either fan the flames of inflammation or promote calm. By focusing on meals free from PUFS and loaded with stable fats instead, you're giving your cells the fuel they need without the irritants. Whether you're just starting to rein in a chaotic gut, or you've been on the healing path for a while, remember that the kitchen is your command center. You dictate what goes in the pan, how it's cooked, and which ingredients make the final cut to your plate.

Sure, habits and cravings can be stubborn. Also, if you're used to the convenience of packaged foods, each adjustment can seem dramatic. But each new dish you master, each snack you reinvent, and each mealtime that leaves you feeling better instead of worse is a step toward transformation. In time, cooking gut-friendly recipes will feel as natural as breathing and far more rewarding than takeout.

—◆—

Mara Makes Low-Toxin Recipes and Posts Them on Social Media

At home, Mara flicked on the stovetop, dropped a pat of ghee into a pan, and watched it melt, hungry for breakfast. As it sizzled, she cracked a couple eggs and added them in. Mara recalled the first time she fried eggs in ghee after reading about how stable it was at higher temperatures. The aroma alone made her mouth water, and the taste was worlds better than any low-fat spray she'd used. This was her new recipe: "Cheesy Egg a la Ghee."

Mara sniggered at the gourmet name she'd created for the simple-yet-delicious meal. In a flash of inspiration, she had the idea to post the recipe on social media.

Yes! she thought. *And then Jake might see it, too.*

Her mind boiled into a thousand fantastical permutations of what could happen when she posted the recipe, all of which ended with Jake cooking the egg dish and loving it. She whipped open her laptop and started to post all of her creations online—the egg dish, and even what Sarah had called her "weird zucchini chips."

The next week, one night at the gym in downtown Chicago, she bumped into Jake. "Hey, I saw you were posting cooking tips online," he said. "I tried the zucchini chips. I made a batch seasoned with sea salt and thyme," his eyes lit up. "They were actually . . . pretty good," he admitted. "And really simple to make, too, which is good for me. I'm not good at cooking. Working on it."

Mara grinned. She should have thought of something clever to say but she just stood there and nodded.

Jake shrugged a little and said, "Well, see you later then."

Even Sarah stepped down from the treadmill to tell her that her new recipes were cool. She hadn't tried any, she said, but it was a cool idea.

Cool. It was cool, Mara thought. Mara left the gym with a spring in her step. Sharing her knowledge felt like sharing some part of herself.

—◆—

CHAPTER 24

Track Your Transformative Journey

One day, not too long from now, you will get up in the morning and your gut will feel fine. No bloat. No scramble for the bathroom. More energy. That is the moment you will realize all your gut-healing effort is paying off. How will you know if that good day isn't a fluke? You will have easy, reliable ways to monitor your progress.

If you're thinking that monitoring will turn you into a data-obsessed scientist, don't worry. You can gain a surprisingly clear picture of what's working and what might need adjusting simply by keeping tabs on everyday symptoms.

The beauty of a good monitoring system is that it respects your body's individuality. No more blind guessing if you're ready for certain foods! By checking in regularly, you'll catch signs that your cells are either happy or in need of a break. Over time, these small snapshots of data offer tangible proof that your approach is on track.

The Belly Speaks Volumes

Symptoms are your gut's version of a text message: They're immediate, unfiltered, and surprisingly specific once you learn the language. The challenge is *not* to brush them aside or assume your symptoms are coincidences. If you wake up and your belly feels like a helium balloon every day, consider that a message.

Energy levels also reveal a part of the story. If you're consistently drained by midafternoon, your cells might not be getting the stable energy they need, or your body might still be dealing with the fallout of PUFS in your meals.

Of course, not every symptom is tied to your gut. Stress from work, a sleepless night on an uncomfortable mattress, and plain old viruses can be contributors. An acute illness—such as a cold or mild flu—can also temporarily spike symptoms, so don't mistake every setback as gut regression. Still, noting how you feel in conjunction with your meals, stress levels, and other variables can indicate which foods correlate with easy-breezy versus meltdown days. Whether you implement some changes or continue on as usual is then your choice.

Gut-Health Journal Template

Monitoring doesn't have to be complex. A basic list in your phone can capture the essence of what's going on. Create a simple "Gut-Health Journal Template" to track your gut health daily or weekly without overwhelming yourself with details. Note morning energy (1–10), gut reactions after meals (bloat, cramping, or relief), mood (feisty or mellow), new foods, and supplements. Mark triggers with an asterisk and checkmark great days.

Don't make it a big deal. Just look for patterns. You may notice that fewer starches resulted in a calmer evening, and postbiotic *Akkermansia* gave you an energy boost. Such insights are great guides toward better gut health.

When to Adjust Your Plan: More than Just a Hunch

The biggest mistake people make is ignoring the signs. Worse, they double down on a strategy that's not working. If your log demonstrates that you haven't been feeling well for several days straight, that's your sign. It doesn't mean your entire approach is flawed; you might just need a minor pivot.

Another time to adjust is when you've felt fantastic for a couple of weeks straight. Why not take the opportunity to expand your menu? If your gut is producing stable stools with minimal bloat, and your energy is on point, you could test a new fiber source or try a slightly larger portion of root vegetables. Your plan isn't carved in stone. Let it evolve as your body gives you new signals.

Check Your Mood and Energy: The Underrated Metrics

Often, gut-health tracking focuses only on digestion: what your stools look like, how your belly feels, and whether you're dealing with gas or cramps. But as we've learned, your gut has a hotline to your brain, your immune system, and your mood. If you've noticed that you're less irritable lately or your brain doesn't fog up as much, your gut could be telling you that its environment is stabilizing. If your mood is all over the place, you might be battling an internal wave of inflammation from daily exposures to irritants.

Monitoring mood and energy can be as simple as rating each day on a scale of 1 to 10. Another option is to use short descriptions such as "focused," "anxious," and "dragging." Over time, you'll see patterns. A stable mental state or feeling more energetic is often the first telltale sign that your gut is turning a corner. That can happen before your digestive symptoms fully calm down.

An important idea to remember is that your cells appreciate consistency. Therefore, don't jump from one extreme diet to another or change up your plan every few days. You won't give your body time to adjust or show you that something is helpful.

Therefore, if your mood is leveling out or your afternoon crash is fading, your body is saying, "Keep going. We like this new routine." Give whatever you're doing more time before shifting or adding something new. Eventually, after you have accumulated numerous green flags, your gut will be able to handle more variety. Likewise, your emotions will better manage stress.

Avoid the Comparison Trap

One of the sneakiest pitfalls in any healing journey is comparing yourself to others. You may see someone on social media claiming they went from a bloated wreck to a marathon runner in two weeks. Why, then, would you still be dealing with flare-ups after a month?

At such moments, you need to stop the comparison game. Everyone's gut is unique, shaped by years of dietary patterns, stress levels, and genetic differences. Healing that takes one person three weeks could require three months for someone else. There's no shame in needing more time.

Your best benchmark is you. That's why your logs, daily notes, and observations are so vital. They anchor you in *your* reality, not someone else's. If you see steady improvements, even if they're tiny, you're on track.

If you and your neighbor both planted tomatoes, and yours were sprouting later, possibly because you had slightly more shade in your yard, would you rip out your garden in frustration? Of course not! You would continue to tend to your soil, pull weeds, and water faithfully. In due course, you, too, would enjoy plenty of fruit.

When the urge to compare creeps in, remember why you began monitoring your results in the first place: to map your personal progress, not to beat someone else's record. Nobody else lives in your body, deals with your schedule, or battles your specific triggers. By staying honest with yourself about the changes you see, you can fine-tune your plan until it genuinely fits you. The goal is a future of not having to give your gut a second thought.

><

Mara Gets an Attitude Adjustment

Mara woke earlier than usual. Golden sun rays broke over the horizon of Chicago buildings. Her mind and body felt refreshed and energized after a long, uninterrupted, restful sleep.

Mara headed to her kitchen for her cup of coffee. Mug in hand, she opened her journal— after months of success with her gut game plan, it sported colorful tabs. Mara diligently entered her observations of positive mood.

The hard evidence was right there in her multi-tabbed journal— her gut was on the mend. Mara pulled on her gym clothes, stepped into her running shoes, and headed for the gym to make it to her strength class on time.

At the gym, there was a new class instructor, Stacey the Bodybuilder. She wore a little orange tankini outfit, showing off her flat, nonbloated belly and smooth, perfectly tanned skin. *Great,* Mara bitterly thought. *Now I have to watch Stacey the Bodybuilder.*

But after class, Stacey stopped Mara with a hand. "Hey!" Stacey smiled with perfect, pearly white teeth. "I hope it isn't too much for me to say, but I follow your recipe page on social media. I think it's totally great!"

Mara blushed. "Really?"

"Yeah," Stacey smiled. "I am always looking for cooking tips. Is it okay if I share your posts a little?"

Mara nodded.

"Great," Stacey beamed. "Well, see you next class."

Mara turned and left. She felt silly for comparing herself to Stacey. She had resented her for no reason. Mara smiled to herself, and now she had another new friend.

CHAPTER 25

Power Your Colon and Fight Metabolic Conditions

Think about how you feel when your energy tanks midafternoon, your pants fit a little tighter, and your energy deflates with a post-meal slump. Such combinations can be the beginning of issues that can lead to problems such as type 2 diabetes and the dreaded label of "metabolic syndrome."

Let's take a close look at type 2 diabetes and obesity, two heavy-weights causing trouble worldwide. You have probably seen many headlines lamenting the rising rates of both metabolic conditions. For years, you probably also heard that the fix is slashing carbs and cutting all sorts of pleasures from your diet. Burning calories, such as by running, possibly sounds familiar as well.

Too often, health professionals ignore the heart-of-the-matter solution: fostering a gut environment that is stable enough to produce ample Gut Gems such as butyrate. When the gut has enough beneficial microbes, they produce plenty of Gut Gems that help your cells manage glucose and insulin more effectively. That means steadier blood sugar after meals, less inflammation, and fewer mid-day crashes.

These common problems would be rare if most people had a healthy gut environment. Instead, burdened by years of PUFS and unhealthy diet choices, modern-day guts can't produce enough of these beneficial compounds.

Mechanisms in Action: Gut Gems Improve Insulin and Burn Energy

Gut Gems such as butyrate shift the body from storing fat to burning it by boosting your cells' ability to use fat for energy and enhancing insulin sensitivity. Butyrate turns on genes that help your mitochondria work more efficiently, reduces inflammation that blocks insulin signals, and triggers hormones such as glucagon-like peptide-1 (GLP-1) that improve how your body responds to insulin.

Improved insulin sensitivity can make or break the fight against metabolic dysregulation. If your cells ignore insulin, your blood sugar stays high. The result is a domino effect that includes fatigue, stubborn weight gain, and an elevated risk of type 2 diabetes. Butyrate helps your muscle and liver cells wake up to insulin's message to let glucose in and use it for fuel. Therefore, you might experience more stable energy after meals instead of that dreaded slump.

Gut Gems also soothe inflammation by calming the immune signals that run wild in a body loaded with PUFS or immersed in chronic stress. By sealing up your gut barrier and telling certain inflammatory markers to settle down, butyrate saves your system from a constant "red alert" mode. When your cells are not stuck in an inflammatory cycle, they can use more energy for everyday tasks such as balancing hormones and maintaining consistent energy.

What the Research Shows

Many of the earliest insights into gut healing came from animal studies, especially in mice. Researchers often fed these mice high-fat, low-fiber diets to induce obesity or inflammation, then supplemented them with butyrate or introduced more butyrate-producing microbes. Across studies, the pattern was clear: These changes led to less body fat, improved blood sugar control, and better insulin sensitivity.

The key? The improvements weren't just from eating less or moving more. The butyrate actually altered the internal environment, boosting energy output, reducing inflammation, and triggering hormones such as GLP-1 that help regulate appetite and insulin function.

These findings suggest that when the gut produces more beneficial compounds such as butyrate, the body shifts out of fat-storing, insulin-blocking mode into a more balanced, fat-burning, insulin-sensitive state.

Human outcomes may not always follow a neat curve, but the overall message is consistent: When you foster a gut environment that produces abundant Gut Gems—especially butyrate—you create the metabolic conditions for real, lasting change.

Once your gut feels ready, gradually adding more fiber back into your diet will also help support your metabolic health in a few different ways. To begin, it slows down digestion and the release of glucose into the bloodstream. This reduces the need for large insulin surges, which in turn improves insulin sensitivity over time.

In addition to the biochemical effects, fiber helps you feel fuller for longer, which often leads to reduced calorie intake. And, as we know, helpful gut microbes feast on fiber and use it as fuel for producing Gut Gems.

Scientific research supports these observations. Many clinical studies and meta-analyses have shown that higher fiber intake improves markers such as hemoglobin A1C (HbA1c, a marker of your average glucose level over the past three months) and fasting glucose in people with type 2 diabetes. Larger studies also consistently associate diets rich in fiber with a reduced risk of metabolic syndrome, type 2 diabetes, and related conditions.

Just remember not to force fiber too early on your healing journey. Stick to the low-and-slow method of reintroducing fiber. Gradually work your way up to a level of fiber intake that works for you.

Gut Gems and Insulin, Show-and-Tell

Each morning, use a glucose monitor to record your fasting glucose level—before eating or drinking anything. If you're using a continuous glucose monitor (CGM), you'll already have this data passively collected overnight. Aim for a fasting glucose level in the 80s, if possible, though your target may vary depending on your starting point.

The Gut Gems–Insulin Connection

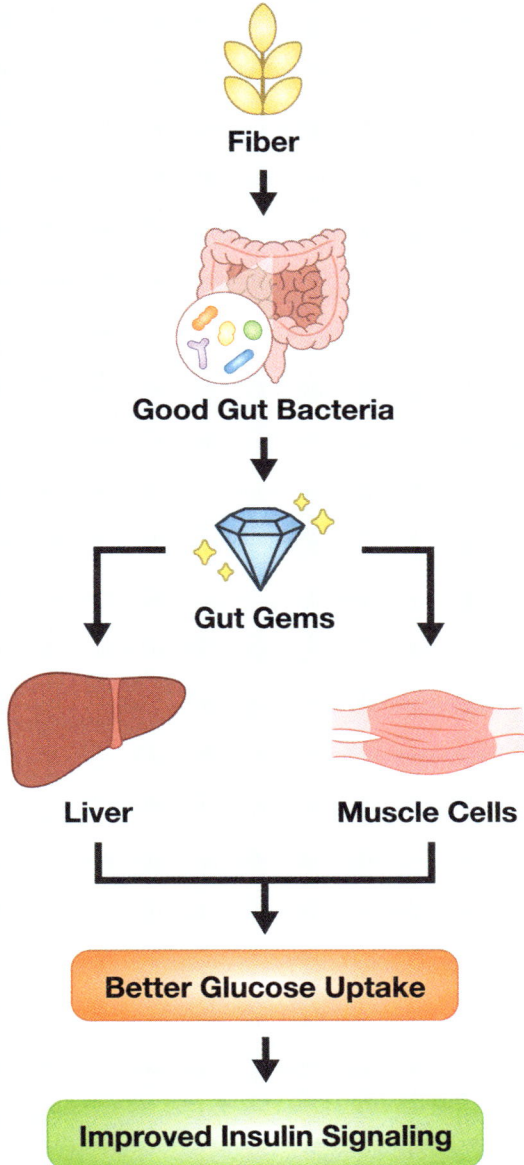

Fiber

Good Gut Bacteria

Gut Gems

Liver   Muscle Cells

Better Glucose Uptake

Improved Insulin Signaling

Fig. 27: Gut Gems travel throughout the body, helping to regulate glucose levels and improve insulin sensitivity.

Then, once or twice during the day, take note of how you feel about an hour after meals—especially your energy, focus, and mood. You don't have to log after every meal. The goal is to notice trends. If you're using a CGM, remember that not all spikes are cause for concern—fruits and exercise can trigger short-term increases that are perfectly normal and physiologic. Don't overcorrect if the context is healthy.

If you're insulin resistant, consider checking your glucose at one and two hours post-meal (with a fingerstick or CGM) to see how long it takes to return to baseline. A spike that stays elevated for more than two hours can signal that your insulin response still needs support. Over time, this gentle tracking method can reveal how your food, gut health, and metabolism are syncing—and where there's still room for improvement.

Celebrate the small wins: a slight drop in your readings and a gentle uptick in your afternoon energy. That's your body telling you, "Hey, this works." If you notice a spike or a crash, examine what may have triggered it. Did you have processed food with seed oils? Could a surge of stress have thrown your hormones off-balance? Your objective is to connect the dots between your daily gut strategy and actual metabolic markers.

Cheering on Your Cells with Butyrate and Gut Gems

When we take a step back and look at the big picture, we can clearly see that metabolic syndrome, type 2 diabetes, and obesity aren't just about counting calories or sweating out an extra mile on the treadmill. Your gut plays a massive role.

Granted, not everyone responds the same way to a new supplement or dietary adjustment. But if you follow the healing paths and strategies we've laid out in this book, you'll likely reap metabolic gains you never thought possible. Nurturing your gut can change your life.

Mara Catches Jake's Attention

Morning sunlight streamed over Mara through a high window at the downtown Chicago gym, spotlighting her as she moved through a deadlift session with focused intensity. Strength surged through her body and her breath flowed in sync with each powerful lift.

Mara no longer relied on mere willpower to get through her deadlifts; she owned a resilient vitality. Mara grinned at her reflection in the mirrored wall.

Mara wasn't the only one to be impressed with her well-earned vitality. Jake noticed her new spark. He gave an approving smile and said, "You're lifting with a different energy these days."

Mara blushed. Jake had never said anything like that to her before.

"You seem happier, too," he added.

Mara watched Jake leave through the front door, speechless. She thought, *Even my social life is doing better since I healed my gut.*

CHAPTER 26

The Gut-Brain Bridge That Shapes How You Think and Feel

We've all had "senior moments"—those times when a name slips our mind or our mood plummets for no clear reason. You might have blamed stress or a lack of sleep. But what if the root cause was deeper, originating not in your brain but in your gut?

Your gut and brain are in constant conversation through a network of nerves, hormones, and immune signals. This communication highway is called the gut-brain axis, and it's increasingly clear that the health of your gut influences how you think, feel, and even remember. When your gut microbiome lacks the right balance of beneficial microbes—particularly those that produce Gut Gems such as butyrate—this internal dialogue becomes distorted. The result? Brain fog, emotional ups and downs, and a decline in resilience.

Growing evidence also links poor gut health to serious neurological concerns, including depression, anxiety, and even neurodegenerative conditions such as Alzheimer's disease. In the pages ahead, we'll explore how butyrate can influence your brain—from helping with mild forgetfulness to supporting the early stages of cognitive decline. You'll also see how rebuilding your gut may help calm those heavy moods that sneak up without warning.

Epigenetic Magic: How Butyrate Talks to Your Genes

Your brain is a marvel, constantly rewiring and adapting in response to life's ups and downs. But it can't work efficiently if the genetic "switches" that direct neuron growth and connections are jammed. That's where butyrate, your favorite Gut Gem, steps in. It can act on your genetic switches through something called histone deacetylase inhibition. To understand the term, think of pressing an "on" button for beneficial genes that might otherwise stay turned off.

Some of these genes are linked to brain-derived neurotrophic factor, better known as BDNF. When BDNF levels are at a healthy level, your brain cells receive the signal to grow, form new connections, and stay resilient. Low levels of BDNF, however, can cause memory gaps and low mood. With enough butyrate around, your body is more likely to keep BDNF production humming and forging a more resilient brain that can bounce back from stress and injury faster.

You might have heard of supplements that boost BDNF. Many articles and books praise meditation and exercise for the same reason. All good points. But if your gut is a train wreck, burdened by PUFS and missing beneficial microbes, your butyrate might be in short supply, which also undermines BDNF.

So, if you were seeking a worthwhile reason to fix your gut beyond avoiding bloating or random belly aches, look no further. A brain equipped with healthy gene expression can keep you sharper as the years roll by.

Taming the Fire: Butyrate's Anti-Inflammatory Shield

You've probably noticed how everyday stress can make your head throb and your mood crash. Why? Your body ramps up inflammatory signals under chronic pressure, fueling a slow, internal burn. While disrupting your gut, inflammation can also seep into your brain, making you more prone to anxious thoughts and mental fog. Over time, relentless stress can chip away at your neurons, raising the risk of depression and neurodegenerative disorders.

Butyrate helps with neuroinflammation, too. Your valuable Gut Gems dial down inflammatory pathways, telling certain cells to tamp down the release of inflammatory chemicals. The shift can help shield your brain from the runaway chain reactions that leave you feeling mentally drained and emotionally on edge. Instead of being stuck in fight-or-flight mode day after day, your system can slip into a calmer baseline.

This doesn't mean you'll never be stressed by the inevitable curve-balls of life, but having sufficient butyrate can help hasten your recovery. If your colon is pumping out enough butyrate, you're less likely to blow a fuse over minor irritations. Also, your mental resilience can stay afloat when bigger storms roll in.

Gut Gems Have a Hotline to Your Brain

As we've discussed, one of the ways butyrate influences your mood and mental state is through the vagus nerve, which connects the gut and the brain. The information exchange travels in both directions. Butyrate enhances communication from the gut to the brain, helping to modulate the stress response.

Gut Gems also play an important role in creating and releasing vital neurotransmitters such as dopamine (pleasure and reward), and gamma-aminobutyric acid (GABA, which promotes optimism, calm, and focus). As mentioned, Gut Gems also promote the expression of BDNF, which then goes on to support the formation of new neurons and the connections between neurons for cognitive and emotional resilience.

Gut Hormones: The Brain's Mood Moderators

Ever notice how certain foods can make you feel instantly better—or worse? Sure, taste and nostalgia are part of that, but your gut hormones also have a say in the matter.

When your gut is balanced, it releases substances such as GLP-1 and peptide YY (PYY) that help regulate appetite, mood, and reward signals in your brain. If your gut is battered by PUFS or starved of the building blocks it needs, you might not get enough of these mood-balancing signals. Gut Gems, especially butyrate, also help maintain the brain's protective barrier by strengthening the cells that seal it shut. Even though only a small amount of Gut Gems reach the brain directly, they still influence brain health by calming inflammation, improving the brain's energy use, and supporting memory and mood from the inside out.

Of course, hormone modulation isn't a quick fix. If your brain has been under the influence of unrelenting stress, poor sleep, and decades of dietary damage, you'll have to do more than pop a capsule of butyrate. In addition, you must support beneficial microbes through the diet and lifestyle strategies we've already discussed. That way, you can build a foundation for balanced hormone signals that flow north to your brain, boosting emotional and cognitive stability.

Gut Gems and Your Brain

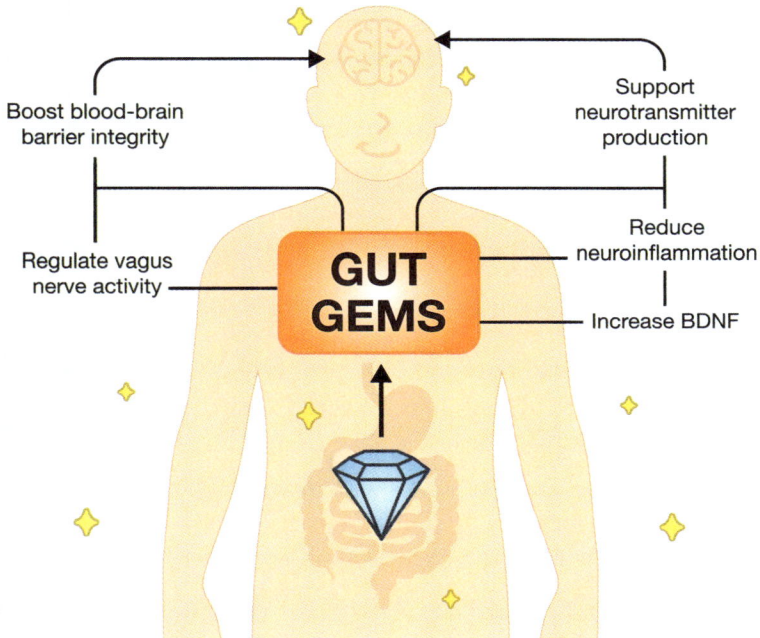

Fig. 28: Gut Gems support your brain and your mental health in multiple important ways.

Energy for Your Brain: Another Trick Up Butyrate's Sleeve

Let's address the mental fog we've all felt at one point or another. Maybe you're on your second cup of coffee, eyes drooping, trying to muster the clarity to tackle a complex task. Brain fog is often a sign that your brain is lacking efficient energy sources. Your brain relies heavily on glucose, but in certain conditions—such as aging or specific health issues—your brain cells can struggle to use glucose well. That's where ketones can come to the rescue, fueling your gray matter even when glucose performance lags.

Butyrate can function like stepping stones for ketones, providing an alternative energy pathway for your brain. If your gut makes enough butyrate, some of it can be converted into the backup fuel molecules that your brain can use. For people dealing with early cognitive decline or fading concentration after certain meals, supporting butyrate production might be the difference between finishing a challenging project and giving up in frustration.

No one is saying you should adopt a strict zero-carb diet or other extreme food restrictions for your body to produce more ketones. The point is that butyrate can help your brain pivot to using ketones when needed. If your gut is brimming with the right microbes (and not burdened by PUFS or toxins), metabolic flexibility becomes more accessible. It is a mental safety net. Mild overnight fasts or post-meal walks can further boost ketone uptake alongside butyrate.

Evidence from Animal Studies

Much of the excitement around butyrate's brain benefits comes from animal experiments. Researchers have run tests on mice with memory issues, anxiety-like behaviors, and artificially induced brain fog. When they introduced extra butyrate or ramped up the microbes that produce it, results repeatedly showed better performance on memory tasks and a calmer response to stress. In some cases, the progression of diseases that mimic Alzheimer's and other cognitive declines slowed.

While mice aren't people, and labs can't replicate your daily routine with all its stress, the animal findings paint a picture of how butyrate might help your neurons adapt. For instance, mice with artificially induced Alzheimer's often accumulate beta-amyloid protein deposits in their brains. Butyrate, by supporting gene expression and reducing inflammation, can lighten that protein load or at least slow its buildup.

Humans are more complex, but the findings in mice make perfect sense: A robust supply of Gut Gems might shield your brain from some of the hits that come with aging or chronic stress. Beyond the memory component, some rodent studies explored mood-related concerns, from anxiety to signs resembling depression. Mice with butyrate support showed better stress resilience and reduced anxiety-like behaviors. Again, while not a direct translation to human psychology, it's an encouraging hint that your gut's production of these compounds can help bolster your mental resilience.

Human Studies: From Observations to Real-Life Trials

When it comes to human biology, the data is a bit more tangled. Our diets differ widely, our stress levels vary from day to day, and we have lifestyle factors that mice in controlled environments don't face. Still, observational research shows a trend: People with less robust butyrate-producing microbes often struggle more with mood swings, mild cognitive impairment, and more serious mental health disorders.

Fecal transplants have also offered glimpses into the power of shifting the gut environment. Folks who receive a new batch of healthy microbes sometimes report better mood or mental clarity, likely because the microbes produce more Gut Gems that calm inflammation and steady hormones. The effect isn't always permanent, though. The gut will revert back to an unbalanced environment if it is continually impacted by PUFS and stress. Nevertheless, the treatments show the potential that lies in rebalancing your colon to tip the scales in favor of mental well-being.

You will hear caution from researchers. Human trials vary: Some are short, some don't use control groups for confounding factors, and others don't isolate butyrate from all the other gut changes that occur. Therefore, one study might praise butyrate for providing a big mood boost, while another claims "not much difference." Real life is messy. Overall, however, evidence supports the idea that a more butyrate-friendly gut helps your brain handle daily ups and downs.

><---->

Mara Goes to Jake's Art Deco House-Warming Party

Mara stood in the middle of the bustling living room at Jake's house, for his dinner party. The vibrant chatter of family and friends hummed around her. Jake hosted a potluck-style housewarming dinner party for his new art deco home on the hill. It was stunning.

Folding glass doors opened to the expansive deck. Mara marveled at the intricate beauty of it, gazing up and all around. Herringbone-patterned wood floors guided her into the dining area, and she noticed that a long, sleek table was filled with bowls of dips, veggie trays, and the usual snack suspects.

Under normal circumstances, Mara would ask polite questions about ingredients. But tonight, who cared! Distracted by Jake, she was off her game. Jake chatted with some of their mutual friends from the gym. He wore a nice suit. She had never seen him in a fine suit like that. At the gym, he always wore shorts and a T-shirt.

A bit flustered, Mara busied herself as he approached; she grabbed a chip and scooped up a heap of creamy dip. Only after placing it in her mouth did the idea of PUFS cross her mind.

"That's my homemade dip," Jake announced. Mara smiled with the chip in her mouth.

"Do you like it?" he asked.

Mara nodded vigorously.

"Good," Jake said, and scooped some for himself.

Unexpectedly nervous around him, Mara grabbed another chip to occupy her hands. Their friends joined in. Crunching away at the chips and dip with everyone else, she felt at ease.

At home hours later, Mara tossed and turned in her bed. Her stomach was bloated and queasy. Her own voice taunted her: *Was it worth it for Jake?*

Mara thought about that. Nothing could be worth this discomfort.

>———<

CHAPTER 27

Butyrate's Anticancer Effects

Gut Gems are powerful allies in the fight against cancer, particularly colon cancer. Over the years, researchers have discovered the many ways butyrate can zap tumor cells or slow their growth. Butyrate performs multiple anticancer functions at once, from editing which genes get turned on or off, to calming the kind of chronic inflammation that invites tumors to grow, to keeping confused cells from turning malignant.

Importantly, butyrate also helps coordinate your immune system, so it doesn't accidentally let cancerous cells set up shop in your colon. That is great news for battling colorectal cancer. Furthermore, since the mechanisms don't always stay quarantined to the digestive tract, other parts of the body can also benefit when the colon is in good shape.

Flipping the Genetic Switch

If you've ever wondered why some cells grow out of control, while others toe the line, it usually boils down to which genes are activated and which are turned down. In a normal scenario, you would want tumor-suppressor genes turned on to instruct suspicious cells to halt or self-destruct. If those genes are shut down, a once-harmless cell might slip into tumor territory. Butyrate can help with that, as it acts as a histone deacetylase inhibitor: It stops certain proteins from silencing the genes that keep cancer in check.

With histone deacetylases blocked, critical tumor-suppressor genes are free to produce the signals your cells need to stay

203

healthy. This shift can trigger apoptosis (or recycling of damaged cells). It could also slow a cell's growth, giving your immune system time to determine if that cell is normal or needs to be removed.

For colorectal cancer cells especially, butyrate's epigenetic nudge is a game changer because it targets the root cause of malignant transformation. That is one reason butyrate has people talking: Not many dietary compounds have such a direct line to gene expression, particularly in a region as prone to disruption as the colon.

Calming the Fire That Fuels Tumors

When people think of inflammation, they often imagine a pounding feeling of a stubbed toe or the body's response to an infection. However, a quieter, chronic version of inflammation can remain in your colon day after day, especially when you have a poor diet. Subtle inflammation can damage cells over time, setting the stage for malignant changes. A body on constant high alert loses the ability to clean up damaged cells efficiently, so a clump of them might evolve into a cancerous growth.

Butyrate can lower inflammation by blocking certain pathways—like NF-κB—that fan inflammatory fires. When your system stops producing so many pro-inflammatory chemicals, your cells aren't battered by daily stress and free radicals. Instead, they're free to do normal cell tasks, such as dividing at a measured pace and dying off when they're supposed to.

For you, that means an environment less hospitable to out-of-control growth—that is, cancer. Think of inflammation as fertilizer for tumor cells. Reducing it starves those cells of the extra chaos they feed on. By helping your gut maintain equilibrium, butyrate makes it harder for malignant cells to flourish. Over the long haul, that can make a real difference in whether suspicious growths get the momentum they need to evolve into full-blown cancer.

Cell Differentiation: Reminding Cells to Grow Up

Cancer often happens when cells refuse to "grow up." Instead of maturing into specialized tissues, they stay in an immature, hyperactive state. Butyrate can prompt these immature or malignant cells to morph back toward normalcy, regaining traits that functional colon cells should have.

For colorectal cancer, that might mean reexpressing markers such as alkaline phosphatase, which helps the cell remember its original function as tissue. Once a cell is forced to differentiate, it's less likely to keep up a crazed proliferation spree. Suddenly the cell starts acting more like a team player, adopting normal growth patterns that don't hog all the resources or spread uncontrollably.

While this isn't a guarantee that every half-cancerous cell will change, if you combine that with butyrate's ability to stifle inflammation and promote healthy gene expression, it lowers the odds of them running rampant. Thus the colon can double- or triple-team the threat and make it harder for a single mutation to form a malignant mass.

Immune Modulation: Rallying Your Body's Defenders

Of course, you're not fighting this battle alone. Your immune system is the bouncer that kicks out unwelcome guests, including cells that decide to multiply beyond reason. However, if your colon is overwhelmed by PUFS, that bouncer can become confused or overburdened, allowing shady cells to slip by. Butyrate helps fine-tune your immune response, promoting regulatory T cells that keep your body from overreacting or underreacting.

The net effect is that your immune cells can better spot suspicious activity without blindly attacking healthy tissues. That's crucial because chronic inflammation is one of the biggest culprits behind malignant transformations. By boosting Tregs— a specialized subset of regulatory T cells that suppress overactive immune responses, prevent autoimmunity, and help resolve inflammation once a threat has passed—and fostering a more balanced immune environment, butyrate ensures your system doesn't inadvertently create a perfect storm for cancer growth. Therefore, while butyrate's strongest effects might be felt in the gut, its influence on your immune system can ripple through your system and offer broader protective benefits.

How Butyrate Protects Against Cancer

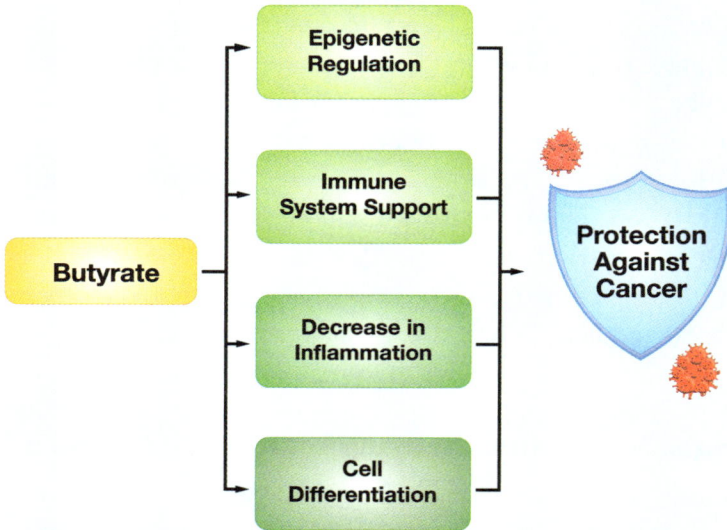

Fig. 29: Butyrate helps keep cancer at bay through multiple important mechanisms.

Cell Studies: What Happens in the Lab Dish

Researchers have evaluated what happens when colon cancer cells are exposed to butyrate in a petri dish. Over and over, they find that malignant cells slow their rate of division, show markers of stress, or kill themselves off. If butyrate can consistently clamp down on malignant traits in a controlled environment, it's worth examining in bigger systems.

That said, your daily life isn't a lab dish. No one is scrutinizing your every meal, ensuring exact doses of butyrate swirl around your colon. You may also have stress, late-night snacks, and occasional dietary slipups with PUFS. Still, seeing the cell-based successes indicates that butyrate has direct anticancer actions at the cellular level, giving hope that a well-tuned gut can replicate some of those benefits in the real world.

Animal Studies: Testing in Mice and Rats

Additional animal studies involving living, breathing rodents provide further insight.

Many cancers, including breast and colon cancer, have at least a study or two suggesting butyrate helps shift the odds in your favor. Mice that receive a consistent dose of butyrate also show inhibited metastasis, meaning the cancer has a harder time spreading to new tissues. From a layperson's perspective, it's incredibly promising. From a cautious angle, we know mice studies are not the same as human trials. The gut flora and stress triggers of mice differ from humans, and they don't have jam-packed schedules or questionable snack habits.

Nevertheless, the animal findings lay the groundwork for why butyrate is taken seriously as an anticancer agent. If a rodent's tumor shrinks or fails to expand when butyrate enters the picture, the indication strongly suggests that controlling your colon environment could lead to similar outcomes. The next logical step, of course, is to see how this all pans out in humans. That is where factors become both exciting and complex.

Human Trials: Spotting Patterns in People

Observational trials suggest a link between diets that foster butyrate-producing microbes and lower colorectal cancer rates in humans. In older studies, typically that meant high-fiber diets. Of course, we now understand the intricacies of fiber. It's beneficial only after you've settled the chaos in your gut and removed PUFS from your diet.

When your gut is stable enough to handle fiber, your microbes can produce more butyrate. Patients who are already diagnosed with colorectal cancer often have fewer butyrate-producing bacteria in their gut, hinting that the shift away from a stable butyrate supply could be part of what allows malignancies to gain ground.

That said, correlation is not proof of causation. This assessment wades through confounding factors—stress, genetics, and lifestyle variables—to be sure. A handful of trials have attempted to give people direct butyrate enemas or tinker with diets to see if colon polyps would shrink or if certain cancer markers would decline.

Results have been a mixed bag. Some show mild improvements, such as reduced inflammation or slower polyp growth, while others remain inconclusive. The reasons vary: small sample sizes, short durations, and the challenge of isolating butyrate's effects in a sea of other dietary and lifestyle factors.

Take, for instance, the idea of using butyrate enemas in folks with ulcerative colitis, which carries a higher risk for colorectal cancer. Some see improvements in gut inflammation and lower cancer risk over time, while others do not see a massive transformation. In other trials, diets aimed at boosting butyrate production led to slight dips in biomarkers that correlate with cancer risk. Overall, the data leans enough on the positive side to fuel ongoing research but not overwhelmingly enough to gain ground in clinical practice.

Potentially, for butyrate to really shine and impact someone's health, it also needs a supportive gut environment: minimal PUFS, a decent stable fat intake that fosters beneficial microbes, and a lifestyle that doesn't continuously sabotage the colon with stress or toxins. If someone is only doing half the job, such as taking a probiotic supplement yet continuing to eat processed foods, the results might not measure up to the success stories from well-controlled studies or lab data.

Butyrate: One of Your Gut's Best Allies Against Cancer

The findings beg the question of what is next for butyrate. We hope to see more research and bigger trials. In the meantime, the takeaway for us is that a gut-friendly routine free of daily PUFS is half the battle. If you can maintain conditions that let beneficial microbes flourish, then your body should produce enough butyrate on its own to mount a decent defense.

While we cannot guarantee a cancer-free life, this strategic move can tilt the odds in your favor. The available research also suggests that, once again, healing and disease prevention start deep in your gut, where the right environment can spark all sorts of protective magic.

Mara Runs into Jake at the Gym

Mara stepped out of her shower, dressed for work, and popped a probiotic supplement into her mouth.

At the zoo offices, she joked about her new energy with her coworker Sasha. "It's a new me, and a new world, and all new doors opening."

Mara wasn't the only one who appreciated her new strength and steady energy. She ran into Jake later that week as she was leaving the gym, and he asked if she wanted to train for a marathon together.

Mara stood there, speechless, and bobbed her head up and down.

"Okay," Jake chuckled. "I'll check in with you later then." As he turned to enter the gym, he ran into the door. Blushing, he shook his head and grinned.

In the following weeks, Mara and Jake trained together. Along with lifting, they ran together and did sprints on the treadmill.

She emerged from the locker room, and Jake was waiting for her. He smiled approvingly and said, "You killed it today! Nice work."

Mara laughed on her way out with him. They were off to grab some smoothies. *It's true,* she thought. *My gut health is improving every area of my life, even my confidence!*

CHAPTER 28

How Gut Gems Can Help You Age with a Smile

Age and chronic disease create a chicken-and-egg situation. Age can rev up chronic inflammation (which the medical research community has termed *inflammaging*), which can increase your risk of all the chronic diseases associated with aging, including heart disease and dementia, as well as stiff knees, aches, and new wrinkles.

As if that's not bad enough, inflammation accelerates the aging process, which can leave you feeling worn out long before the years have racked up. The more Gut Gems you produce (or the more butyrate you get, if you need to supplement), the more you can tamp down the fires that flare up in your cells.

If your gut has a decent handle on making Gut Gems, your cells will be better able to dodge some of that inflammatory burden that creeps up with each birthday. You might not feel like you've cheated old age entirely—after all, there's no magic potion—but you could add to your health span, meaning the number of years you spend in good health, free from chronic disease or disability.

No one wants to spend their retirement years battling poor health. Aging well doesn't mean staying invincible but rather reducing the daily wear and tear that can make getting older feel harder than it has to be.

Why a "Longevity Lifestyle" Really Matters

Some people stay vital into their nineties and beyond. You

may chalk it up to good genes, but the real secret behind their healthy longevity more likely stems from the day-to-day habits that keep them active, engaged, and less burdened by chronic inflammation. Sure, genetics play a role, but your daily choices contribute tremendously. If you keep eating PUFS, skimp on sleep, and blow off managing your stress, you're essentially inviting the inflammaging process to speed up. Keeping your gut robust enough to produce Gut Gems is a big piece of the "longevity lifestyle" puzzle. So, if you'd like to feel well through-out your older years, consider the following changes:

- **Daily diet:** Replace PUFS with stable saturated fats. That shift alone can lift a load off your system. Also make sure you're getting enough protein each day—adequate protein intake helps preserve muscle mass and prevent sarcopenia as you age.

- **Movement:** You don't have to run marathons, but the bene-fits of consistent activity such as daily walks or dancing add up to something meaningful. Gentle movement can stoke your overall vitality, so your gut doesn't stagnate, and your entire system stays more balanced.

- **Social connections:** Social connections are often over-looked, but laughing with friends, chatting with a neighbor, or having a Zoom call with family can have a surprisingly calming effect on your gut. If you want to keep your internal environment as friendly as possible, find ways to stay con-nected. It can be as valuable as any supplement out there.

- **Stress:** Too much stress sets your immune system on edge, and a stressed gut produces fewer Gut Gems.

When you combine these lifestyle adjustments, you end up with synergy to help your cells work more smoothly, letting you enjoy life on your terms. The real win is waking up one day realizing you feel more vibrant than you did last year and knowing you're taking steps to extend that feeling of vitality and health as long as you can.

Gut Gems Benefits Timeline

Sometimes motivation peaks when you see the finish line—or at least an outline of where you're headed. That's where a timeline of Gut Gems benefits comes in handy. This simple chart maps out what might happen in the short term, the medium range, and the long haul if you consistently nurture your gut. In the first few weeks, for instance, maybe your bowel habits become more regular, or you notice you're no longer struggling with post-meal bloat. Another month or two down the road, you might see improvements in your energy levels or clearer skin.

Fast-forward a year or two and you might be looking in the mirror and seeing a more vibrant version of yourself, and feeling less weighed down by day-to-day annoyances. The timeline below isn't a list of strict deadlines. Every human body has its own rhythm. The schedule is more of a friendly reminder that real change takes time, and the best results don't happen overnight. Each step you take to boost Gut Gems is an investment in how you'll feel down the road.

What to Expect as Your Gut Heals

Timeline	What You Might Notice
Weeks 1–4	Bowel habits begin to normalize. You may feel less bloated, have more regular digestion, or feel relief after eating. Meals might feel less daunting.
Months 2–3	Energy levels become more stable throughout the day. Skin may look clearer. You may feel lighter and less sluggish after meals.
Months 4–6	Inflammation markers may lower, and subtle joint stiffness might ease. You may notice sharper thinking, fewer afternoon crashes, and improved resilience to stress.
Months 7–12	Better immune response (fewer colds), smoother movement, deeper sleep. You might feel less emotionally reactive and more in sync with your body's cues.
Years 1–2	A renewed sense of vitality. Your skin, digestion, and focus all feel more balanced. You feel more "yourself"—less burdened by discomfort or fog.

Fig. 30: The benefits of focusing on your gut health continue to grow over time.

Bringing It All Together: A Happier Future Awaits

I want you to maintain your zest for life—and your ability to enjoy it—as you age. So, you can't ignore what's happening in your gut. Without taking mindful steps to counteract inflammation, it can sap your energy, interfere with your focus, heighten stress, and challenge you to care about all those wonderful details that make life worth living.

Thankfully your gut has a natural shield against this downward spiral—those beloved Gut Gems. That's not to say you can wave a magic wand and watch your wrinkles fade. Real health is layered, and your gut is just one (very important) piece of the puzzle. A well-tuned gut can give you a spark of youthful energy that lasts a lot longer than you'd expect.

In the end, it's not about obsessing over every bite or even measuring your success by how many years you can tack on to your life. It's about how good you can feel right now, how gracefully you can navigate the decades ahead, and how much joy you can squeeze out of each day. That said, here's to your future. May it be filled with calmer days, sharper mornings, and a gut that rewards you for taking care of it!

＞━━━＜

Mara, Sarah, and Stacey the Bodybuilder Go to the Spa

Stacey sat with her feet in a small salt-soaking tub. Mara and Sarah each had a white mask peel covering their faces, so they looked like mummies, or lucha libre wrestlers, or something. Out the window, autumn leaves swirled in the wind.

Mara let out a great groan and reclined onto the wood bench of the spa sauna room. "Work at the zoo has been insane. So much stress. Hate the orangutans lately."

"At least that sounds like a fun job," Stacey admitted glumly. "Bodybuilding is tough. It feels like I'm never enough sometimes. At least going to the spa and this type of thing helps. I always worry that the stress of it all is pushing my body too far. It ages me."

Mara propped her head back up. "You know that might be true. Our lifestyle influences the way we age, more than we think.

The biggest factors are stress, diet, and movement. Funny enough, social connections impact how we age, too."

"That's why when we're ninety I'll still be cracking jokes at you," Sarah poked, talking through the gap in her face mask.

"Not me," Mara brushed her off and adjusted her own mask. "I'm never aging at all. I'm keeping my diet top-notch. Might need to find some new friends, though."

"Hey!" Sarah teased back, and swatted Mara. And the two of them pushed back at each other in a type of flapping, slapping pretend fight.

"I wish the two of you knew how ridiculous you looked," Stacey sniggered. "Like two mummies fighting."

"But these two mummies will age gracefully, won't we?" Sarah said, hooking Mara through the arm.

Mara nodded and rested her head on Sarah's shoulder. And for the first time in a while, she felt at home.

><del></del>

CHAPTER 29

Emerging Research on Gut Gems and Gut Health

Regardless of everything we've covered regarding gut health, new research comes out every day. The rapid leaps in knowledge represent a lifeline of hope for anyone struggling with a gut-related condition. In this chapter we'll look at some of the most recent and exciting research that shows the therapeutic powers of Gut Gems.

Gut Gems Are Key for Gastrointestinal Health

Gut Gems are an important defense against all kinds of gastrointestinal maladies. For example, inflammatory bowel disease (IBD) triggers intense gut inflammation, but boosting butyrate and other Gut Gems can help restore balance. In diabetes, when metabolism becomes unstable, research shows these molecules help steady blood sugar levels. In chronic kidney disease, a well-balanced gut microbiome can indirectly support kidney function. It's a remarkable feedback loop—the gut supports whole-body health, and in return, your body helps maintain a healthy gut.

Recent research also underscores butyrate's pivotal role in aiding recovery from infections affecting the gastrointestinal tract. A study published in *Microbiology Spectrum* revealed that patients with Clostridioides difficile infection (CDI)—better known as C. diff—had significantly reduced levels of Gut Gems, especially butyrate, compared to healthy individuals.

Butyrate also turns down the fire of autoimmunity by attaching itself to T cells, which are regulatory immune cells. Butyrate activates the T cells, which can then call off rogue immune cells that would otherwise attack healthy tissue. Without butyrate, the T cells slack off and chaos can erupt.

Gut Gems Keep Your Neurons Happy

Another aspect of health where butyrate plays a powerful role is in the brain. Impressive evidence exists to suggest butyrate's benefits to brain health. Adding a tasty pat of butter to your food, therefore, includes neuro insurance. Also, remember that PUFS are easy targets for oxidation, and that fuels inflammation. Therefore, swapping them for saturated fats avoids inflammation before it starts.

Regarding the research, a 2018 study published in *Frontiers in Immunology*, conducted at the University of Illinois, found that giving butyrate to older mice reduced inflammation in brain immune cells (microglia). The results support the idea that butyrate may help brain health by lowering inflammation, possibly through boosting antioxidants such as glutathione.

Butyrate has also been found to increase levels of brain-derived neurotrophic factor (BDNF), which cues the formation of new neurons as well as new connections between existing neurons. Butyrate boosts BDNF by blocking the enzymes that turn down BDNF genes.

A 2018 study published in *Frontiers in Aging Neuroscience* investigated the effects of probiotic and prebiotic supplementation—thereby increasing butyrate production—on cognitive function in middle-aged rats. According to the findings, the treatment significantly improved spatial memory in a maze task (Barnes maze) and increased hippocampal BDNF levels while reducing pro-inflammatory cytokines.

In March 2025, *Frontiers in Aging Neuroscience* published a study that evaluated data from the extensive National Health and Nutrition Examination Survey (NHANES) conducted from 2011–2014. It found that older adults (age sixty and up) who ate more butyrate had better brain function.

A 2025 report in *Ecological Genetics and Genomics* found that people with Alzheimer's disease have a distinctly different mix of gut bacteria compared to those without the condition. Using data from 176 individuals, researchers discovered that Alzheimer's patients had higher levels of certain bacteria like *Phocaeicola*, *Bacteroides*, and *Faecalibacterium*, while levels of *Avispirillum* were lower.

This microbial imbalance is thought to play a role in worsening Alzheimer's by disrupting the gut-brain connection, increasing leaky gut, raising inflammation throughout the body, and reducing beneficial compounds, such as butyrate, that help protect brain function.

The findings add to growing evidence that your gut and brain are closely linked. This study suggests that gut health may be a promising target for future Alzheimer's treatments and early detection tools. Early studies in mice with Huntington's disease also show that giving them butyrate helps improve movement problems and even helps them live longer.

Microbiome Transplants and Gut Gem Infusions

When your gut gets wiped out—by antibiotics, chronic illness, or inflammation—you may need more than just a probiotic. Sometimes your gut needs a full reboot. That's where microbiome transplants and targeted Gut Gem therapies come in.

Fecal microbiota transplantation (FMT) works like a reset button for your gut. Doctors take a full spectrum of healthy gut bacteria from a screened donor and transfer them to someone whose microbiome has been badly damaged. This approach has shown powerful results for stubborn infections like C. diff, allowing healthy bacteria to crowd out the bad ones and start producing beneficial compounds such as butyrate again. In some people with ulcerative colitis, FMT can also reduce symptoms and help heal the gut lining, especially when those transplanted microbes boost butyrate production.

In cases where inflammation affects just the lower part of the colon—like ulcerative proctitis or radiation damage—butyrate enemas offer another way to deliver relief. These treatments aim to directly restore Gut Gems to the affected tissue. Results have been mixed, often because people find the nightly routine hard to stick with, but the potential is there. Whether through transplant or targeted delivery, these therapies highlight a simple truth: Sometimes healing your gut means restoring the ecosystem that makes it work.

A 2017 study in *The Lancet* looked at eighty-one patients across three hospitals in Australia. It found that 27 percent of those who received FMT went into remission from ulcerative colitis, compared to just 8 percent in the group that didn't get the treatment.

For several years, nanotechnology has been used as a delivery system in research. A 2017 study in the *World Journal of Gastroenterology* reported that coadministration of dexamethasone, a synthetic corticosteroid (more powerful than natural cortisol) plus butyrate by nanoparticles could be beneficial for inflammatory bowel disease treatment.

In a 2024 study published in *Bioengineering & Translational Medicine*, scientists created a special probiotic called EcNP3 that was engineered to produce propionate. When they gave the probiotic to mice with colitis, the animals' symptoms improved. The treatment worked by balancing the gut bacteria and reducing harmful immune reactions.

If you're curious about participating in a microbiome transplant trial, visit the ClinicalTrials.gov website, search for "butyrate" plus your condition, and scan the map for nearby trials.

Research Roundup

Here are three additional research papers that offer a glimpse of the many powerful benefits of Gut Gems.

1. A January 2025 study published by *Nature Metabolism* showed how propionate and butyrate attach to proteins called histones, which help control which genes are turned on or off. This shows how your diet directly affects your metabolism and the way your genes behave.

2. A 2025 study in *Pharmacological Research* found that specially engineered yeast may help protect the heart from damage during cancer treatment—and it does so by working through your gut. Radiation therapy often harms healthy tissues, including

the heart. In this mouse study, researchers discovered that yeast designed to produce butyrate not only helped maintain the intestinal barrier and reduce gut inflammation after radiation but it also protected heart tissue from radiation damage. The yeast worked by restoring a key gut receptor, boosting helpful microbes such as *Akkermansia* and *Lachnospiraceae*, and enhancing the body's use of compounds such as taurine and nicotinamide. This chain reaction led to the activation of heart-protective genes that reduced inflammation and tissue damage. By reinforcing the gut-heart connection, this research points to a new way to reduce the side effects of radiation—potentially protecting not just your heart but other vital organs as well.

3. A 2024 study in *Gut Microbes* found that gut bacteria that produce butyrate are significantly reduced in people with gastric cancer. When mice received transplants from these patients, they developed more tumors—unless they were given butyrate, which boosted cancer-fighting CD8+ T cells. This protective effect relied on a key gut receptor, highlighting the potential for butyrate-based therapies to help prevent or manage gastric cancer by restoring immune strength through the gut. While mouse studies don't always translate directly to humans, findings like these offer promising clues about how gut-based therapies could influence immune function and cancer risk.

Staying on the Cutting Edge

Staying informed about emerging research can be empowering. You don't need a PhD to keep up. Let's break down two ways you can stay informed.

The first way is to set aside a little time each month to see what new research has come out in the world of gut science. You can find quick summaries of new discoveries online. Blogs will sometimes translate scientific jargon into plain English. A lot of news outlets provide simplified explanations, which is all you really need to see if there's something relevant to your life. Reliable places to start include *ScienceDaily* and *Medical News Today*, both of which feature summaries of the latest research written for everyday readers.

If you want a deeper dive, you can go straight to PubMed (pubmed.ncbi.nlm.nih.gov). This website is hosted by the National Library of Medicine and it warehouses research published by medical journals. You can search for "butyrate" or "short-chain fatty acids" and add the year to locate the latest papers.

The AI platform Perplexity is another great place to search for studies. Here, you can simply ask, "Please find the latest studies on short-chain fatty acids" (or ask for the latest studies on butyrate). In addition to hyperlinks to the studies in question, you'll also receive a short description of each.

You might read about a new study that ties high levels of certain microbes to better mental clarity. Or you'll see that scientists have discovered a new microbe that helps regulate your appetite. Such updates help you connect the dots and consider if anything resonates with your gut struggles. The bottom line is you don't have to become an expert. Just staying in the loop makes you less likely to fall for outdated diets and questionable quick fixes.

Stay-Curious Challenge

Another approach is to make a game of being informed. Commit to reading at least one gut-related study or article each month. Give yourself gold stars or checkmarks if that kind of motivation helps. It might sound silly, but hitting small goals can keep you from drifting off into the land of "I'll do it tomorrow." Over time, you'll build a solid stash of knowledge while connecting the dots between your daily habits and the broader science of how your gut thrives or struggles.

Maintaining an attitude of curiosity also guards against hype. If you hear about some brand-new gut miracle that "cures everything," you'll know enough to question whether that's possible. Knowledge keeps you grounded. Each bit accumulates and shapes a more confident, proactive approach to looking after your body.

━━━━◄

Mara Learns How to Use PubMed and Realizes It's Not That Hard

The kettle hissed. Steam fogged a nearby windowpane, lighting the pink hues of dawn in a dreamy effect. During enchanted autumn mornings like this, Mara loved living in a Greystone townhouse. In her kitchen, Mara whipped open her laptop and searched for Gut Gem studies on PubMed.

How sophisticated I am, Mara thought, smugly. *I must be smart. I must really be something.*

The old Mara would never do this. She had demanded quick fixes. She had thought of herself as a victim. But the new Mara was here.

Mara sipped her green tea and scrolled deeper into the findings of a fresh meta-analysis on the ability of short-chain fatty acids to reduce inflammation and promote healing in gut disorders such as colitis. The news was good. The butter she had swirled into her tea (instead of the vanilla-flavored, PUFS-filled creamer she used to use) really did have the potential to help keep her painful inflammation at bay.

But gut health wasn't the only thing she searched for. Aunt Linda had slipped into early dementia. Too many casseroles, maybe, but who knew . . . Mara bit her lip, scrolling through articles. This really wasn't so tough, this whole PubMed thing. This whole research thing. She could take the future of health into her own hands. She could learn almost anything.

━━━━◄

CHAPTER 30

Innovations in Gut Microbiome Testing

Thanks to recent developments in gut microbiome testing, doctors and scientists can now dive deeper into the specific environment in your gut. A new testing mechanism called "high-throughput sequencing" allows labs to run detailed tests on thousands of microbes at once. That means cheaper, faster, more accurate tests that can give you a clearer snapshot of what's happening inside your gut.

Are your microbes in good shape? Is your gut pumping out enough butyrate to keep your immune system at peace? Beyond just how much and what kinds of bacteria and Gut Gems you *have* on hand, cutting-edge tests might soon reveal if your gut cells are able to *use* the Gut Gems you have to strengthen the lining of your gut.

There's also growing interest in assessing how Gut Gem levels influence cognitive symptoms such as brain fog and mood swings. By testing your personal microbiome, you get a peek behind the curtain. Therefore, you can make adjustments to support your mental health.

Having this level of insight into what's going on in your gut is a game changer. For instance, your microbial profile could seem pretty normal on paper, but if the synergy between your microbes and your gut cells is off, you may still end up with a leaky gut. Verifying that the synergy is happening—or not—is crucial for deciding whether you need a different diet strategy, or another approach entirely.

Why This Matters for Your Everyday Life

By finding out where your system stands, you can address the real issues instead of diving headfirst into the next fad diet. Understanding the latest innovations in gut testing can allow you to be more strategic.

Just remember that advanced tests won't fix your gut. You can pour over all the data, but committing to a new plan for your health is what will give you results. Meaningful progress comes when you pair knowledge with action.

The Future of Gut Testing

Soon enough, we might see a world where a simple at-home kit tells you exactly which microbes in your colon need extra support and which ones are producing butyrate. That might sound futuristic, but practical tools are closer than you might think.

Another development on the near horizon is wearable health technology that can track your microbial balance and Gut Gem levels in real time. The devices, particularly when paired with AI-driven recommendations, are set to revolutionize personalized gut-health management.

While no mainstream wearables currently measure Gut Gems, several innovations are in the works, such as ingestible smart capsules that travel through the gastrointestinal tract and measure temperature, pH, and the presence of certain gases such as hydrogen and methane that can correlate with gut dysbiosis. As of right now, these are only research prototypes. There are no consumer devices available yet.

Research is also underway to develop wearable biosensors, such as skin patches, which can detect microbial metabolites in sweat or breath. Potentially an app will one day give you real-time dietary and behavioral advice based on the information detected by wearables.

The possibility for crossover between gut tests and wearables is heightened by AI, which can synthesize and analyze data from multiple sources—such as microbiome test results, dietary logs, sleep data, and mood tracking. As a result, you could receive a comprehensive understanding of how your gut-brain axis is functioning.

In the next few years, we can expect to see AI also use this information to predict which interventions—such as prebiotics, probiotics, or types of fiber—will most effectively reduce symptoms. And it could update the predictions based on changes in what you've eaten or how you've slept.

With the right testing, you will gain a road map. With the right road map, you will make better decisions. With better decisions, you will be on the road to a healthier gut and a better life—one that isn't constantly sabotaged by hidden inflammation or misguided dietary advice.

If you're wondering whether gut testing makes sense for you, the short answer is *maybe*. Not everyone needs an in-depth analysis. However, if you're fed up with guessing and want real clarity on how to help your colon, the new testing techniques are worth a look. They're becoming more accessible, more user-friendly, and more tailored to regular people like us.

Keep your curiosity alive and remember that knowledge is only as good as how you use it. If you decide to use it, you can rest assured that gut science can lend a helping hand.

─────

Mara Faces the Ultimate Test

A brown paper–wrapped package arrived one morning at Mara's front door. It was a new gut microbiome test she had ordered in the mail. No doctor was needed; she could test herself and send in her results right from home. It was a new type of stool test that claimed to measure actual butyrate levels.

When she had first heard about it, she wanted to dismiss it as more hype, but her curiosity got the better of her. Although the test was still new, she loved that she could see concrete evidence of her progress that would prove that she had locked in a healthier gut.

Months ago, if she had known how easy and affordable these tests were, she would have started here, to understand her baseline. Maybe she would have saved herself months of guesswork and self-doubt—or maybe not. Would she have been too stubborn to take the tests? Early on, probably yes!

She pulled the box in and set it on the kitchen counter. For her, the promise of real-time feedback set her at ease. It was somewhat like tracking macros or recording personal bests at the gym.

Mara wound down for the evening and recorded a quick note in her journal: "I've arrived at real change, and I can see how it's all tied together—my diet, my training, my sanity. I'm living it."

><

CHAPTER 31

Personalized Nutrition: Your Custom Gut GPS

You made it through the trenches. You banished PUFS, embraced saturated fats, and got your Gut Gem production back on track. Your belly is feeling so much better. It's time to bring in a post-healing menu that suits your needs, your gut, and your preferences. In other words, you're ready to personalize your nutrition by choosing foods that crank out more Gut Gems, soothe leftover inflammation sparks, and match your microbiome right now.

Your microbiome is like the weather—changeable and occasionally dramatic—so you should adapt what you put on your plate accordingly. Staying attuned to your gut health means there is no "forever diet." What works one week may not work as well the next. Personalized nutrition gives you tools to adjust without panic.

Your Personalized Nutrition Plan

To tailor your diet to your gut, start by taking a gut assessment, whether that's a basic at-home stool test or a clinical panel.

Next, keep a simple food intake and symptom journal. Just make quick notes of what you ate and how you felt—from bloating, to energy, to skin glow. Aim for seven days of baseline data. During that time, eat as you normally do before making any changes to your food choices, supplements, and lifestyle practices.

Once you have a week of data, assess it to see if certain foods produce predictable results. Some will likely be good (more energy, better sleep, no bloating). Some might be bad (cramps, bathroom troubles, mood dips). Based on your findings, adjust your meals accordingly.

Custom Diet Builder: Cracking the Code on What Your Gut Needs to Flourish

The first time you open a microbiome report, the colored bar graphs and Latin names might be confusing, possibly overwhelming. To create your own personalized nutrition plan, you need only rely on three insights:

1. The top five beneficial species

2. The top two or three unfriendly strains

3. Your overall diversity score—or how many different strains you're hosting, keeping in mind that the more diversity you have, the more resilient your gut is

Knowing the results helps you make choices. For instance, if *Bifidobacteria* are low, lean on banana-flour pancakes or green-tipped plantains. When you have sufficient *Bifidobacteria* to munch on prebiotic carbs, they can churn out Gut Gems and vitamins such as folate.

If *Akkermansia* is low, sprinkle in pomegranate-peel powder or cranberry juice shots. Both can boost the mucus lining that *Akkermansia* loves to nibble on.

To translate your test results into a plan, choose one gut bacteria that your test results suggest you're lacking and research its favorite snack. Add that particular food three times in the next week. Note how you feel after consuming it to determine how it may be affecting you.

Your symptoms matter more than any generic recommendation. If, for example, your test results show that you are low in the bacteria *Prevotella*, it may suggest eating black beans to nurture these gut microbes. Well, if you know black beans make you uncomfortably gassy, don't force yourself to eat them. You could try an alternative instead, such as ripe kiwi or kiwi-fiber powder. Ease in foods slowly and retest later. Personalized means adjusting, not suffering.

Likewise, remember that your gut may not be ready for large amounts of fiber foods. Start with small portions of easily digested carbs, such as mashed ripe plantain, stewed apples, cooked carrots, and overnight oats soaked until soft. These foods are more likely to ease their way through the GI tract without triggering a lot of gut distress while still giving your microbes the carbs they need to produce Gut Gems.

Meanwhile, keep PUFS off the menu. Watch out for salad dressings, granola bars, and crackers. They gum up mitochondrial gears and slow Gut Gem production. Replace them with saturated fats: butter on your overnight oats, coconut oil–roasted sweet potatoes, and dark-chocolate squares. Aside from specific foods that will suit your microbiome, consider how much of each macronutrient— protein, carbs, and fats—your body needs. For most people, a balanced starting point might look like 30 percent fat (mostly saturated), 15 percent protein, and 55 percent carbohydrates from real food. Others may feel better with a slightly higher fat intake—40 percent fat, 15 percent protein, and 45 percent carbohydrates—especially during times of healing or metabolic repair.

That said, your sweet spot may be different and vary from day to day depending on how well you slept, how active you are during the day, and if you're getting over an illness. Feel free to experiment and keep an eye on which proportions feel best for your body.

An easy reference for getting adequate protein is to aim for a palm-sized piece at each meal. Protein supplies amino acids that repair the gut lining and keep cravings at bay. Bonus: Many proteins— including oysters, red meat, shellfish, poultry, and eggs—come with zinc and iron, the minerals that fuel enzymes that turn Gut Gems into anti-inflammatory messengers.

When it comes to carbs, the more physically active you are on a given day, the more you tend to need. On strength-training days, add baked yams. On desk-job days, stick to carrots and berries. The ebb and flow keeps glycogen tanks topped without inviting a post-meal energy crash.

Micronutrients matter, too. Magnesium acts as the key in over three hundred enzyme locks, including ATP synthase (your cell's energy bank), and helps regulate bowel movements by relaxing smooth muscle in the colon. Vitamin D modulates immunity, so your gut wall doesn't treat every crumb as an invader. Sprinkle seared salmon with cilantro-lime salt, chase with a shot of full-fat kefir, and voilà—you get magnesium and vitamin D in one tasty swoop.

Testing, Tracking, Tweaking

To keep tabs on how your personalized nutrition plan is panning out, schedule a monthly check-in. At this time, weigh yourself, measure your waist circumference, and take a selfie of yourself in natural light (no filters) to gauge your skin clarity and overall vitality. If you love data, give yourself an inexpensive finger-stick test that measures your C-reactive protein (CRP) level—an inflammatory marker that can indicate how well you are removing PUFS and sugar. The ideal hs-CRP range for healthy adults is less than 1.0 mg/L, which indicates a low risk of cardiovascular disease and minimal underlying inflammation. A level between 1.0 and 3.0 mg/L indicates a moderate risk, and anything above 3.0 puts you in a high-risk category.

If you want, do a gut microbiome test once a quarter to see if you need to shore up any specific bacteria and assess how well your dietary changes are impacting your Gut Gem productions. Remember, microbes adapt to what you feed them. As you nail down what works for you, that's great, but don't eat the same foods repeatedly. Why? A diversity of food sources promotes a diversity in the microbiome.

>———◄

Mara Gets an Inspired Idea

Mara opened her food journal and read the prior day's notes that she had scribbled in violet ink: "Less bloating after plantain mash; afternoon energy 8/10."

Just as she flipped to a fresh journal page, ready to chart that day's notes, her laptop chimed. The results of her stool test were in. She took a screenshot of the highlights and dragged them into her notes app. Apparently her *Bifido* was low. She'd have to change that. She wrote herself a reminder to make banana-flour pancakes for breakfast the next morning, a natural source for *Bifido*. She stuck it on the fridge door where she wouldn't miss it. And she made a mental note that starting off the day with carbs would help her prepare for her planned lunchtime workout.

Before bed that night, Mara completed an at-home CRP test; it was one of the personalized tests she had committed to use. She sealed the kit and set it by the door to mail the next morning. The results would take a few days, but she had hope. Everything else in her routine, including other test results, pointed to progress on her journey to optimal health.

Pride rippled through her. If she had created these achievements for herself, she could help others do the same. An idea surfaced in her mind, and she sent off a quick email to the gym owners:

> Hi Bethany and Thomas,
>
> This is Mara. I had a fun idea. Would you be open to the idea of me hosting a potluck meal at the gym? Besides being a fun event, it would be a great opportunity for me to pass along some amazing things I have learned about gut health. I promise to arrange everything. What do you think?
>
> Mara

CONCLUSION

The Path to Gut Health

You've made it to the end of the book, and that's worth celebrating. If your journey so far has felt like a series of ups and downs, know that this is normal. Gut health has twists, and you've navigated them like someone who refuses to settle for "just okay." Such drive will continue to power you forward!

Do you remember when you first learned how toxins could wreak havoc on your digestion? Did you have any idea how much the invisible troublemakers could mess with your gut? Then you learned about butyrate, the star Gut Gem that helps patch up your colon and keep those toxins from sneaking through. That was a big revelation! Your gut can't do much with fiber if the environment is riddled with damage in the first place. People love to talk about vitamins and minerals, but butyrate often stays in the background. All the while, it's quietly running the show.

If toxins have left your gut barrier in a sorry state, butyrate swoops in with reinforcements, sealing up the cracks so that the environment becomes friendlier. Only then does it make sense to bring fiber back into the mix. As you now understand, if your gut is under siege, piling on fiber can just stir up more chaos.

Healing, of course, doesn't happen overnight. Sure, you may feel better after a week or two of focusing on butyrate, ditching the PUFS that irritate your cells, and adding gut-friendly snacks made with butter or coconut oil. But for deeper healing, you'll need to be consistent. That's not always the most exciting message. Who wants to hear "be patient" when you're feeling unwell? Yet patience is often the key that unlocks real transformation. When you slowly nurse your colon back to health, focusing on real nourishment day after day, you give your cells the time they need to rebuild a sturdy gut lining. Now you also know that the body is interconnected, so a calmer gut can lead to calmer everything.

Your Future Starts Today

At this point, you might be itching to put all of this into practice, or maybe you're still on the fence, wondering if it'll actually work for you. Here's the truth: Nobody else can walk this path for you. The encouraging news is that you don't need a complete life overhaul on day one. Sometimes the best progress comes from a single small step that sparks confidence and momentum.

The biggest hurdles usually aren't the changes themselves but the mental resistance you might feel. Changing old habits can be tough, especially if you've been told for years that you need to fear fats or that fiber is the only path to digestive salvation.

Despite that noise, you can trust your gut—literally and figuratively. Your gut has an incredible capacity to bounce back, especially when you remove irritants and give it the nourishment it craves. You're aiming for real, long-term healing that's going to serve you well beyond the next few months. And guess what? Your cells are more than ready to jump on board. They just need the right environment to do their job.

If you find yourself hesitating, think of how much better life might be when you're not pinned down by gut drama: more energy, more spontaneity in your meals, and fewer nights spent cradling a bloated belly. That's worth pushing through the initial discomfort of trying something new. Yes, it can feel odd to unlearn old habits or stand by your new choices when friends and family question them. But if you keep the vision of a healthier, happier gut in mind, your internal motivation can propel you further than any amount of peer pressure can hold you back.

Take a Gut-Health Pledge

Making a gut-health pledge is your opportunity to draw a line in the sand. It begins with a simple statement, such as, "I promise to give my gut a fighting chance by prioritizing healing and nourishment."

It might sound corny, but you'll be far more committed when you put your intentions into words. Write it down and put the pledge where you'll see it every day. Your refrigerator might be a great place. You want that reminder that you're not just reading about gut health but *living it*.

The pledge becomes real when it includes a specific action. Therefore, you might decide to say, "I pledge to take a probiotic supplement daily" or "I pledge to cut out PUFS for the next three weeks." Pick a concrete action that aligns with your gut's needs. This is *not* a punishment. It's the gift of a happier, healthier future.

Don't worry if you stumble. Quite frankly, you should prepare yourself for slipups. They won't mean you've ruined everything. If you simply forget (or try to ignore) your pledge, you're human! Acknowledge that it happened, reboot, and keep going.

The real power of any pledge lies in what you do most of the time, not in being perfect every single second. Over time, the vow you make to yourself will become second nature, and that's when you'll notice that your gut has genuinely begun to transform.

Give Yourself a Gut-Health Hero Certificate

If you started making changes well before you got to this point in the book, congratulations are in order! The Gut-Health Hero certificate is a lighthearted way to recognize how far you've come. After all, you've navigated the complexities of toxins, discovered the role of butyrate, tackled PUFS, and learned why timing matters with fiber. That's a lot to take in, so why not mark the accomplishment?

You can design a simple certificate on your computer or on paper. The real value is in the moment you step back and say, "Hey, I did something big here."

Your certificate can be just for you or something you share with loved ones who might also be on a gut-healing journey. If you have a friend who's been reading along with you, the two of you can swap certificates and celebrate the steps you've taken. Don't underestimate the power of camaraderie. Knowing that someone else appreciates what you've gone through—reading, learning, shifting your habits—can make your progress feel more satisfying. Plus, it affirms that you're not just passively learning; you're actively championing your cells to feel better.

Simply looking at your certificate can trigger you to keep going. For that reason, hang it where you'll see it often, maybe near your pantry or wherever you've placed your pledge. Both will remind you that you have a choice every single day about what you put into your body and how you nurture your gut. That can give you the boost of confidence you need when you're debating if it's worth making coconut oil–based snacks instead of grabbing a PUFS-filled bag of convenience.

A Final Note on Small Steps

Remember, healing is the sum of a thousand little choices you make each day. Think about it: Every climber who reached the summit of Mount Everest did so by taking one step at a time.

Over weeks and months, your individual decisions can reshape your entire digestive landscape. As a result, you will notice changes in how you feel. With less bloating, steadier energy, and a calmer mindset, you will want to continue to honor your gut's needs. One day you'll realize you've built a whole new routine around healing.

As you close this chapter, give yourself a moment to soak in the fact that you've stuck with this, diving far deeper than most people ever do. Most importantly, you've seen that a better gut is possible. You can achieve lasting results, and you now have the tools to make that happen.

———✦———

Mara Hosts a Potluck

Mara closed the hatchback of her car and carefully balanced a steaming dinner dish of chicken and veggies cooked in ghee. The afternoon potluck at her downtown Chicago gym was on!

Mara grinned at the idea of how far she'd come. *Just months ago,* she thought, *my diet was hijacked by PUFS-filled convenience foods and secondhand nutritional advice.* Now she was about to host the gym's first-ever gut-health potluck. Her heart fluttered with excitement.

Mara entered the gym and saw the familiar faces of her friends; Sarah, Jake, Stacey, and so many others showed up. She'd once considered it a place to "out-lift" and "outrun" her digestive woes. Her gut was a battleground back then, yet she had no idea what it was fighting. Through curiosity, dedication, resilience, and patience (well . . . mostly stubbornness at first), Mara finally had a whole squad of friends by her side to cheer on her long-term health and happiness.

Jake broke her train of thought as he approached the potluck table with a bowl of stir-fried vegetables. He proudly announced they were cooked in coconut oil instead of his usual canola oil. "I'm learning from you," he said with a wink.

Mara's cheeks became hot. She felt a flash of humility and a bit of amazement all at once. Perhaps now she was a mentor, a guide for those who were ready to follow the path of self-ownership for their health.

The dishes that lined the table were every color and every kind of food. In preparation, Mara had drafted a basic, one-page "cheat sheet" for everyone that featured three phases.

Remove PUFS.

Prioritize butyrate.

Reintroduce fiber gradually.

The path seemed obvious to her now. It had all become so second nature to her. She had no question that coaching her friends was the most natural and helpful thing she could do. And an idea dawned on her: She could become a full-time gut-health coach. *Yes! That's it!* she thought.

On her way home, her heart turned with excitement at the prospect of helping others transform their lives.

As she crawled into bed that night, Mara relaxed fully into the soft sheets. Her gut was strong, and her mind was made up. With all she had learned and accomplished, Mara was ready to lead others with confidence and, most importantly, compassion.

><

Appendix: The Science Behind *Gut Cure*

One of the core strengths of *Gut Cure* is its foundation in rigorously documented science. This section includes the simplified version of the original paper that forms the backbone of the book's research. This version is designed for everyday readers who want to grasp the big-picture insights without getting lost in molecular pathways or technical jargon.

This transparency is intentional. It reflects a core principle of the scientific method: You should be able to evaluate evidence firsthand, not just rely on expert interpretation. Whether you're a curious reader or a seasoned clinician, having access to the full body of research empowers you to think critically and draw your own conclusions.

That said, science doesn't stand still. This paper, like this book, reflects our best understanding at the time of writing. But as new studies emerge and technologies evolve, our knowledge will continue to grow.

Short-Chain Fatty Acids Influence the Gut-Brain Connection—Simplified Paper

Abstract

Background: Short-chain fatty acids (SCFAs) are small fatty molecules—such as acetate, propionate, and butyrate—that are made by bacteria in the colon when they break down dietary fiber. These molecules act as key intermediaries in the interactions between diet, gut microbes, and the human body as a whole. SCFAs affect the health of both the gut and the brain. This scientific review looks at how SCFAs function in the communication network between the gut and the brain, known as the gut-brain axis. Within this gut-brain system, SCFAs support colon health by fueling colon cells and strengthening the gut's barrier. At the same time, SCFAs that enter the bloodstream can influence how the nervous and immune systems interact (neuroimmune pathways). They also affect metabolism and cognition. Over time, our diets have changed dramatically: Our ancestors ate plenty of fiber (around 50–150 grams per day), but modern Western diets only provide about 15–20 grams per day. This shift from a high-diet fiber to a low-diet fiber has greatly reduced the production of SCFAs, and this is associated with an unhealthy imbalance of gut microbes (dysbiosis), inflammation, and an increase in chronic diseases such as colorectal cancer, metabolic syndrome, and neurodegenerative disorders. SCFAs normally help counteract those problems by inhibiting enzymes called histone deacetylase inhibitors (HDACs), thereby reducing inflammation, increasing the numbers of regulatory T cells (Tregs; cells that keep the immune system in check), and controlling appetite. However, modern Western diets—high in omega-6 fats and artificial additives—make the SCFA shortage even worse.

Purpose: There are several strategies aimed at restoring SCFA levels to fix gut-brain axis problems. These strategies include:

- **Prebiotics,** which are indigestible fibers (like inulin or resistant starch) that feed healthy gut bacteria
- **Probiotics,** which are beneficial live bacteria that can be ingested

- **Direct SCFA supplementation,** such as giving butyrate through enemas

- **Fecal microbiota transplantation (FMT),** which transfers gut bacteria from a healthy donor into a patient

Challenges include optimizing treatment delivery and encouraging broad adoption. This review combines historical background, biological mechanisms, and practical insights to assert that SCFAs can help restore a healthy balance within the gut microbiome and improve health.

Introduction

Short-chain fatty acids (SCFAs) are a type of fat molecule with fewer than six carbon atoms. The major examples of SCFAs are acetate (C2), propionate (C3), and butyrate (C4). These SCFAs are recognized as crucial mediators in the complex relationship between diet, the microorganisms in the gut, and the body. SCFAs are mostly produced by obligate anaerobic bacteria (bacteria that can't survive in oxygen) in the colon. The bacteria create SCFAs by fermenting dietary fibers that are not broken down earlier in the digestive tract.

In a healthy human colon, the SCFAs acetate, propionate, and butyrate are usually found in roughly a 60:20:20 ratio (about 60 percent acetate, 20 percent propionate, and 20 percent butyrate), and each plays a distinct role. SCFAs have two main kinds of effects on the body. Locally in the gut, they keep the colon healthy and act as the main energy source for colon cells. Systemically (throughout the body), they have metabolic and neuroactive effects that can even influence how the brain works. The term *gut-brain axis* describes the two-way communication network between the gut and the central nervous system (the brain and spinal cord). In this gut-brain network, SCFAs are important signaling molecules. They can influence pathways that link the nervous and immune systems (neuroimmune pathways) and might even affect behavior and cognition.

Modern lifestyles and diets, however, may be disrupting this ancient mutually beneficial relationship we have with our SCFA-producing gut bacteria. The rapid shift in the past century from fiber-rich traditional diets to the low-fiber Western diet has caused a drop in SCFA production in our gut. Concurrently, modern populations have been eating an abundance of certain fats, especially linoleic acid (LA), an omega-6 polyunsaturated fat (PUFS) common in highly processed vegetable oils and seed oils. These dietary changes are thought to contribute to gut microbial imbalances (dysbiosis) and an increase in chronic inflammatory and metabolic diseases. That is why it is crucial to understand the role of SCFAs in our health and how our diet affects the production of these molecules.

This review explores various strategies to restore optimal SCFA levels. These include changing dietary practices—such as increasing fiber intake and modifying fat consumption—as well as through direct SCFA supplementation and delivery methods. It evaluates how these approaches affect gut dysbiosis and inflammation and considers current challenges in using SCFAs as therapies. Throughout the article, historical context, biological mechanisms, and practical applications are examined with the goal of supporting better individual health outcomes.

Gut Microbes and SCFAs in Gut Health

The human gut microbiota (the microbes in our intestines) is largely made up of anaerobic organisms (oxygen intolerant). In the colon, these microbes ferment complex carbohydrates that are not digested earlier in the intestine. They produce a wide array of enzymes to break down plant polysaccharides (complex carbohydrates from plants), including fibers such as resistant starch, inulin, pectin, and cellulose. The microbes convert these into simple sugars and short-chain compounds, which are then further metabolized into SCFAs. These bacteria are obligate anaerobes, which thrive in the colon's low-oxygen (hypoxic) environment that is maintained by colon cells that consume any available oxygen. As a result, eating a diet high in fermentable fibers encourages a gut microbial community full of SCFA-producing species. In other words, what we eat (especially fiber) is closely tied to the SCFAs our gut microbes produce.

Early studies culturing gut bacteria revealed that the colon is densely populated with bacteria that are largely anaerobic. Bacteria in the colon outnumber human cells by about ten to one. Later research confirmed that about 99 percent of colonic bacteria are obligate anaerobes. The most common groups of bacteria in this community are from the Firmicutes and Bacteroidetes phyla. In particular, Firmicutes include many Clostridia (such as species in the *Roseburia*, *Eubacterium*, and *Faecalibacterium* groups), and Bacteroidetes include bacteria such as *Bacteroides* and *Prevotella*. These bacteria utilize special enzymes (glycoside hydrolases and polysaccharide lyases) that break down complex plant carbohydrates that the body cannot digest. The low-oxygen environment of the colon makes it an ideal place for fermentation. These findings built a solid framework for understanding the microbial ecosystem behind SCFA production in the human colon.

Key SCFA-Producing Bacterial Genera and Their Preferred Substrates

Bacterial Genus	Primary SCFA Produced	Preferred Substrates	Notable Functions
Faecalibacterium	Butyrate	Resistant starch, complex polysacs	Anti-inflammatory, high abundance in a healthy gut
Roseburia	Butyrate	Inulin, arabinoxylan	Promotes mucosal health and synergy with other fermenters
Bacteroides	Acetate, Propionate	Wide range of polysaccharides	Versatile saccharolytic capacity, common in Westerners
Eubacterium	Butyrate	Starch, fibers, cross-feeding	Cross-feeds on lactate/acetate, is beneficial for colon health
Anaerobutyricum hallii	Butyrate	Lactate, acetate, some starches	Potential probiotic candidate, has synergy in butyrate production
Bifidobacterium	Acetate, Lactate	Oligosaccharides (FOS, GOS, HMOs)	Often early colonizer in infants, cross-feeds to butyrate production

Table 1: Key short-chain fatty acid (SCFA)–producing bacterial genera, their primary SCFAs, preferred substrates, and notable functions, illustrating microbial contributions to gut homeostasis.

Within the colonic environment, SCFAs are absolutely essential for maintaining intestinal balance (homeostasis). Butyrate especially is the main energy source for colonocytes (the cells lining the colon). It provides about 60–70 percent of the energy these cells need by fueling their mitochondria, where fatty acids are broken down (a process called beta-oxidation) to produce adenosine triphosphate, or ATP, the cells' main energy source. This energy support helps maintain a healthy colon lining (mucosa) and strengthens the gut barrier. Butyrate promotes the formation of tight junctions (the seals between cells) and stimulates the production of mucus and antimicrobial peptides (short proteins), which are key defenses that reinforce this barrier.

SCFAs also play a powerful role in preventing colorectal cancer, a phenomenon sometimes called the "butyrate paradox." In healthy colon cells, butyrate is a crucial fuel that supports cell health. However, in colon cancer cells, which rely on a different energy process, butyrate is not used as fuel and instead builds up. In those cancer cells, the accumulated butyrate inhibits histone deacetylase (HDAC) enzymes, causing the cancer cells to stop dividing and to undergo programmed cell death (apoptosis).

Population studies strongly link high-fiber diets with a lower risk of colorectal cancer. Animal studies support that link: in rodents, adding extra fiber to the diet or delivering butyrate into the colon via enemas reduces tumor formation. Scientists are increasingly interested in new strategies to prevent colorectal cancer that involve butyrate, such as using probiotics that produce butyrate or using methods to deliver butyrate directly to the colon. These approaches could serve as preventive treatments (chemoprevention), especially for people at high risk of colon cancer—such as those with hereditary polyp conditions—and offer a promising path forward in colorectal cancer prevention.

The immune-modulating role of SCFAs raises theoretical concerns in certain cases, such as advanced cancer (where suppressing the immune system might be risky). However, overall, SCFAs are known more for their protective effect against colorectal cancer by supporting a healthy epithelium.

From Gut Microbial Imbalance to Future Therapies: Molecular Pathways

Beyond their crucial role in colon health, SCFAs act as key regulators in the gut-brain axis. The gut-brain axis is a complex two-way communication network between the gut environment and the central nervous system. Of all the SCFAs produced in the colon, a small fraction (about 5–10 percent) is absorbed into the bloodstream and travels to the liver via the portal vein. Acetate is the most likely to reach the rest of the body because colon cells use up most of the butyrate, and the liver removes most of the propionate. Only a small portion of SCFAs in the blood can cross the blood-brain barrier (BBB) through specific transporters. Even so, SCFAs that enter circulation can have widespread effects. They influence neural, immune, and hormonal pathways, which in turn can affect brain function in important ways.

SCFAs can affect the nervous system both directly and indirectly. For example, acetate acts on nerve pathways in the gut lining; it sends signals that influence circuits in the hypothalamus (a part of the brain) that control feelings of fullness and energy expenditure. Propionate, another SCFA, stimulates specialized cells in the gut lining (enteroendocrine L cells) to release hormones such as peptide YY (PYY) and glucagon-like peptide-1 (GLP-1). These hormones reduce appetite and send "full" signals to the brainstem and hypothalamus. Studies in humans support this mechanism: When the colon produces more propionate, people tend to eat less and gain less weight. In rodents, propionate and butyrate make the body more sensitive to leptin (a hormone that suppresses appetite) and activate pathways that reduce hunger. This protects the animals from diet-induced obesity and insulin resistance, highlighting the role of SCFAs in regulating metabolism.

In addition to these benefits, SCFAs also support brain health. They reduce inflammation (which is a contributor to depression) and support proper neural function, which can positively affect mood and cognition. SCFAs can influence neurotransmitter systems, help regulate the hypothalamic-pituitary-adrenal (HPA) axis, and strengthen the BBB—making them crucial mediators in the gut-brain axis and helping explain how an unhealthy gut can lead to neuropsychiatric issues.

SCFAs also have strong effects on the immune system, indirectly influencing the brain. They reduce inflammation throughout the body, and by doing so, they affect how the central nervous system functions. When SCFA levels are high, they strengthen the gut barrier, making it less "leaky." This prevents harmful substances like lipopolysaccharide (LPS an endotoxin from certain bacteria) from passing into the bloodstream. By keeping LPS out of the blood, SCFAs help reduce metabolic endotoxemia (the presence of endotoxins in the blood, which can trigger low-grade, chronic inflammation) and stop the chain reaction of inflammation that can affect the brain. Maintaining the gut barrier, along with promoting anti-inflammatory immune cells (such as regulatory T cells in the colon and IL-10-secreting macrophages in the circulation), creates an immune environment that is less likely to trigger inflammation in the brain.

Moreover, SCFAs can affect the body's stress-response system: the hypothalamic-pituitary-adrenal (HPA) axis. In animal studies, extra butyrate blunted stress-induced HPA activity and led to less anxious behavior. Studies comparing germ-free mice (which have no gut microbes and thus no SCFAs) to normal mice show that SCFAs help calm the stress response. These endocrine (hormonal) effects highlight SCFAs as important regulators of the balance between the nervous, immune, and endocrine systems.

Gut microbes also produce various neuroactive compounds, and dysbiosis (microbial imbalance) can reduce their production. For example, certain *Bifidobacteria* produce gamma-aminobutyric acid (GABA), a calming neurotransmitter. When *Bifidobacteria* are depleted due to dysbiosis, less GABA is made in the gut, meaning fewer calming signals reach the nervous system. Butyrate also has effects within the brain by inhibiting HDAC enzymes in the central nervous system. This epigenetic effect (changing gene expression without altering DNA) increases the production of brain-derived neurotrophic factor (BDNF), a protein that enhances brain plasticity, learning, and memory. SCFAs can also directly affect brain cells. For instance, acetate can alter how the brain recycles neurotransmitters such as glutamate and glutamine, and butyrate boosts BDNF levels through epigenetic mechanisms. Together, these mechanisms link diet, microbial metabolism, and brain physiology–making SCFAs

Gut-Brain Axis Communication by SCFAs

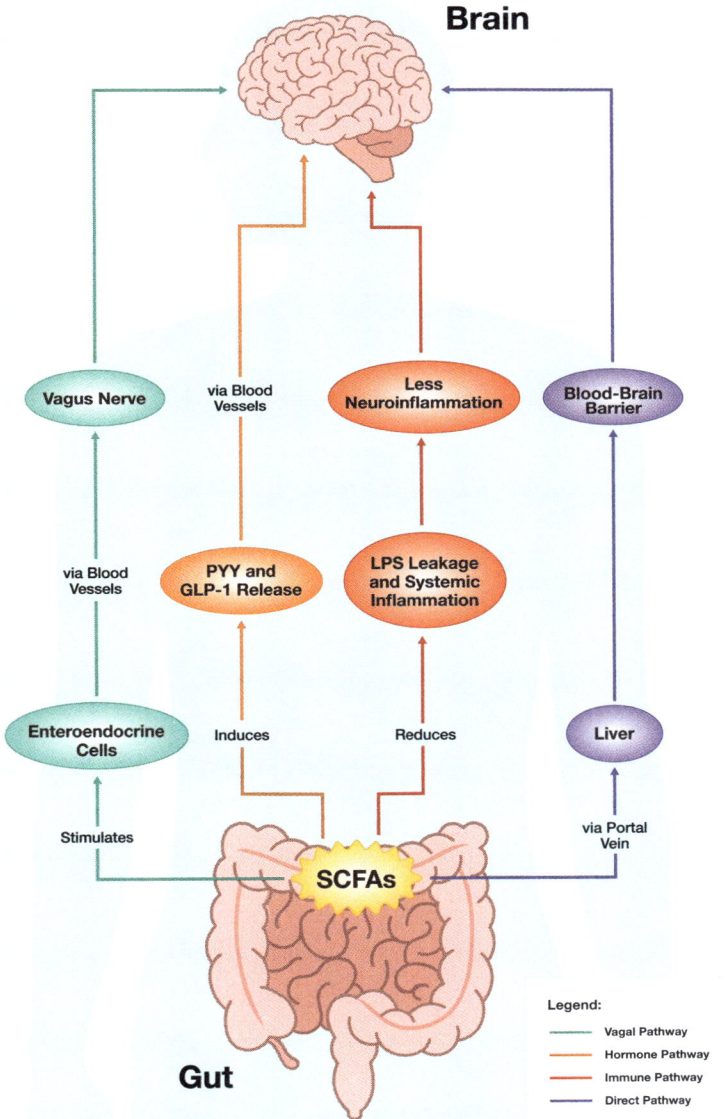

Fig. 31: Illustration of the gut-brain axis communication mediated by short-chain fatty acids (SCFAs), depicting pathways through which SCFAs influence neural, metabolic, and immune functions.

a critical linchpin. Disruptions in SCFA signaling are increasingly implicated in neurodevelopmental disorders, mood disorders, and neurodegenerative diseases.

SCFAs as Key Factors in Both Ancient and Modern Health

SCFAs exemplify the complex biochemical partnership between our diet, our gut microbiome, and our body's functions. In early human populations, diets were very high in a variety of plant fibers. These fiber-rich diets supported a diverse community of fermentative bacteria in the gut, which produced plentiful SCFAs. Consistently high SCFA levels in those ancestral diets likely helped promote a tolerant immune system (one that doesn't overreact) and kept metabolism in balance. These SCFAs may even have played a role in how the human brain evolved by signaling through the gut-brain axis over millennia. Unfortunately, modern industrialized diets—full of refined foods, low in fiber, and filled with chemical additives—have greatly reduced SCFA production by our gut microbes. This is a fundamental departure from the diet our bodies evolved to eat, leaving the modern public in an SCFA deficit with broad health implications.

Contemporary Western diets are very different from traditional high-fiber diets. Traditional diets often included over 50–100 grams of fiber per day, whereas the modern Western diet provides only about 15–20 grams. For example, present-day hunter-gatherers such as the Hadza of Tanzania still eat around 80–150 grams of fiber daily from tubers, fruits, and wild plants—highlighting how fiber-poor modern diets are. In the United States, the average person consumes only about 16 grams of fiber per day, far below the 25–38 grams recommended. This major shortfall in fiber means SCFA-producing gut bacteria don't get enough fuel. As a result, those bacteria produce far fewer SCFAs, weakening the overall gut ecosystem.

Exacerbating the lack of fiber, Western diets are full of components that negatively reshape our gut microbiome and metabolism. Eating an abundance of omega-6-rich fats and refined sugars encourages the growth of bile- and acid-tolerant microbes (such as certain *bilophila* species and members of the Enterobacteriaceae family) at the expense of fiber-fermenting bacteria. This shift leads the micro-

**Changes in Gut Microbiota from
Traditional High-Fiber Diets to Western Low-Fiber Diets**

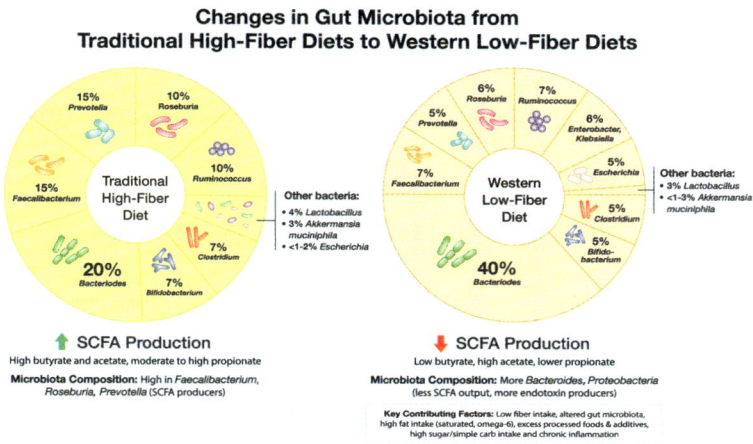

Traditional High-Fiber Diet

- 15% Prevotella
- 10% Roseburia
- 10% Ruminococcus
- 7% Clostridium
- 7% Bifidobacterium
- 20% Bacteriodes
- 15% Faecalibacterium

Other bacteria:
- 4% Lactobacillus
- 3% Akkermansia muciniphila
- <1-2% Escherichia

↑ **SCFA Production**
High butyrate and acetate, moderate to high propionate
Microbiota Composition: High in *Faecalibacterium*, *Roseburia, Prevotella* (SCFA producers)

Western Low-Fiber Diet

- 6% Roseburia
- 7% Ruminococcus
- 5% Prevotella
- 6% Enterobacter, Klebsiella
- 7% Faecalibacterium
- 5% Escherichia
- 5% Clostridium
- 5% Bifido-bacterium
- 40% Bacteriodes

Other bacteria:
- 3% Lactobacillus
- <1-3% Akkermansia muciniphila

↓ **SCFA Production**
Low butyrate, high acetate, lower propionate
Microbiota Composition: More *Bacteriodes, Proteobacteria* (less SCFA output, more endotoxin producers)

Key Contributing Factors: Low fiber intake, altered gut microbiota, high fat intake (saturated, omega-6), excess processed foods & additives, high sugar/simple carb intake and chronic inflammation

Fig. 32: Comparative pie charts illustrating shifts in gut microbiota composition and SCFA production between traditional high-fiber diets and Western low-fiber diets, highlighting microbial and metabolic changes.

biome to produce more endotoxins and fewer SCFAs. Additionally, processed foods often contain emulsifiers, artificial sweeteners, and preservatives that disrupt gut microbe function. For example, dietary emulsifiers (such as carboxymethylcellulose and polysorbate 80) can erode the gut's protective mucus layer. In animal studies, consumption of dietary emulsifiers led to gut inflammation, driven by changes in the microbiota. Common artificial sweeteners such as saccharin and sucralose have been shown to cause dysbiosis and alter SCFA profiles in both rodents and some human studies. All these additives, combined with environmental pollutants that enter the food chain, further suppress SCFA production.

Building on this, other substances commonly encountered in the modern world can also act as "mitochondrial toxins," damaging the mitochondria, the energy centers of cells. These toxins can include dietary pesticides, excessive alcohol, and other food-borne contaminants. They may directly impair how colon cells use butyrate for energy and disrupt microbial fermentation pathways. Environmental pollutants such as dioxins and polychlorinated biphenyls (PCBs), which accumulate in animal fats, can also damage mitochondria across tissues. Long-term exposure to these toxins harms the gut-lining cells (enterocytes) and microbial metabolism. If colon cells use fewer SCFAs due to mitochondrial damage, there may be less feedback to support butyrate-producing bacteria, further reducing butyrate. In other words, this breaks the mutually beneficial nutrient exchange between us and our gut microbes. All these factors together—lack of fiber, harmful additives, and mitochondrial stressors—combine to attack gut homeostasis. The result is dysbiosis characterized by lower SCFA levels and a weakened microbiome.

The "Vicious Cycle" of Fiber Deficiency, Dysbiosis, and Mucus Layer Degradation

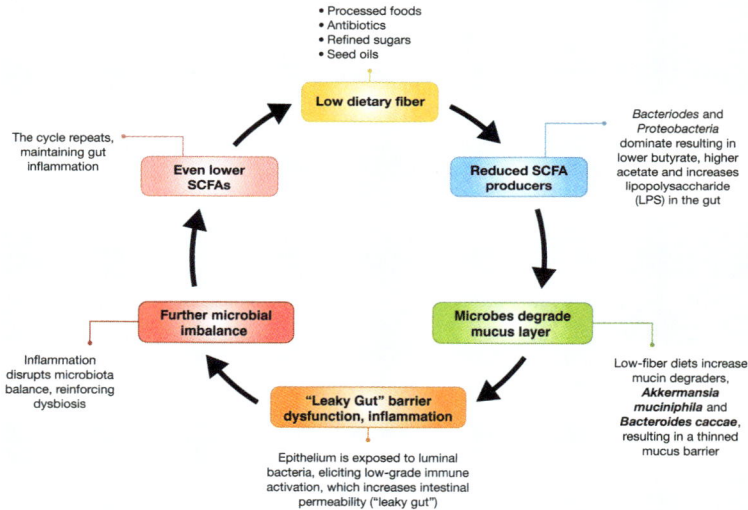

Fig. 33: Schematic representation of the vicious cycle linking low dietary fiber intake to reduced SCFA production, microbial dysbiosis, and mucus layer degradation, perpetuating gut inflammation and barrier dysfunction in Western dietary patterns.

Why Low SCFA Levels Matter: Effects on the Gut-Brain Axis

A decline in SCFA production doesn't just affect the gut; it has far-reaching effects on the whole body. In the colon, if there are not enough SCFAs (especially butyrate), colon cells lose their main energy source. This energy shortfall can lead to the colon lining becoming weaker or even shrinking (atrophy), and the gut wall becomes more permeable (leaky gut). Clinically, low fecal butyrate levels are strongly associated with inflammatory bowel diseases (IBD) such as ulcerative colitis and Crohn's disease. Early clinical trials show that targeting the gut microbiome can modulate SCFA pathways. For example, a trial in ulcerative colitis patients using a microbiome-based therapy achieved moderate remission rates and seemed to increase patients' own SCFA production.

In fact, giving SCFAs directly (especially butyrate enemas) has been shown to improve mild ulcerative colitis, underlining how important butyrate is for healing the gut lining. Systemically, not having enough SCFAs can lead to metabolic problems. In animal models, supplementing diets with butyrate or propionate helped prevent obesity from a high-fat diet and improved insulin sensitivity by enhancing satiety signals and increasing energy expenditure. In humans, metabolic syndrome (a cluster of conditions including high blood sugar and excess body fat) often occurs alongside a dysbiotic gut microbiome that is low in SCFA-producing bacteria. Early human trials show that adding fermentable fiber to the diet or using SCFA-mimicking compounds can improve blood sugar control and reduce body weight.

The Discovery of SCFAs: Historical Insights into Gut Fermentation

Scientists first identified SCFAs as important products of gut microbes in landmark studies of intestinal fermentation in the nineteenth and early twentieth centuries. The first SCFA discovered was butyric acid, isolated in 1815 by the French chemist Michel Eugène Chevreul from spoiled butter (the name *butyric* comes from the word *butter*). It was later found in human feces, providing early evidence that gut microbes produce fatty acids.

A key breakthrough came in 1966 when Robert E. Hungate performed a lab experiment using human fecal samples to ferment dietary fiber. He showed that the main fermentation products were acetate, propionate, and butyrate. This finding established that gut microbes ferment carbohydrates to get energy, producing SCFAs in the process. In the 1960s and 1970s, the advent of gas-liquid chromatography (a lab technique used to separate and quantify chemical compounds) allowed precise measurement of SCFAs in fecal samples.

This made it possible to directly link what people ate to the SCFA profiles in their gut.

Around the same time, scientists studying ruminant animals (like cattle and sheep) provided insights into human SCFAs. In cows, fermentation in the rumen (a part of their stomach) produces an abundance of acetate, propionate, and butyrate. Researchers found that high-grain diets in these animals shifted fermentation toward propionate, while fiber-rich forage diets produced more acetate and butyrate—changes driven by shifts in microbial populations. Even though the human colon differs from a cow's rumen, these findings established an important principle: Diet determines what metabolites gut microbes produce. This concept—that diet shapes microbial metabolite production—remains key to understanding human gut health.

Fiber-Rich Diets and Low Disease Rates

Mid-twentieth-century research revealed a striking contrast: Populations eating traditional diets high in fiber and low in processed fats and sugars had far lower rates of chronic diseases than those in industrialized populations. The pioneering doctors Denis Burkitt and Hugh Trowell, working in East Africa, observed that rural communities there rarely experienced conditions such as appendicitis, colon cancer, or heart disease. They attributed this resilience to the fiber-rich diets of these communities. These observations formed the basis of the "fiber hypothesis," which proposes that dietary fiber is key to preventing many Western diseases.

Burkitt and Trowell mainly focused on fiber's mechanical benefits, like bulk to stool. However, their work also hinted at the role of the gut microbiota: In high-fiber diets, gut bacteria ferment fiber into SCFAs, which have protective effects. Modern science shows that SCFAs are multitalented regulators. They not only maintain the integrity of the colon lining but also modulate lipid metabolism, keep the immune system in balance, and support blood vessel function—largely by reducing inflammation and helping stabilize blood pressure. Thus, the historically low disease rates in high-fiber populations may be mechanistically linked to elevated SCFA levels that suppress inflammatory pathways and keep metabolism stable.

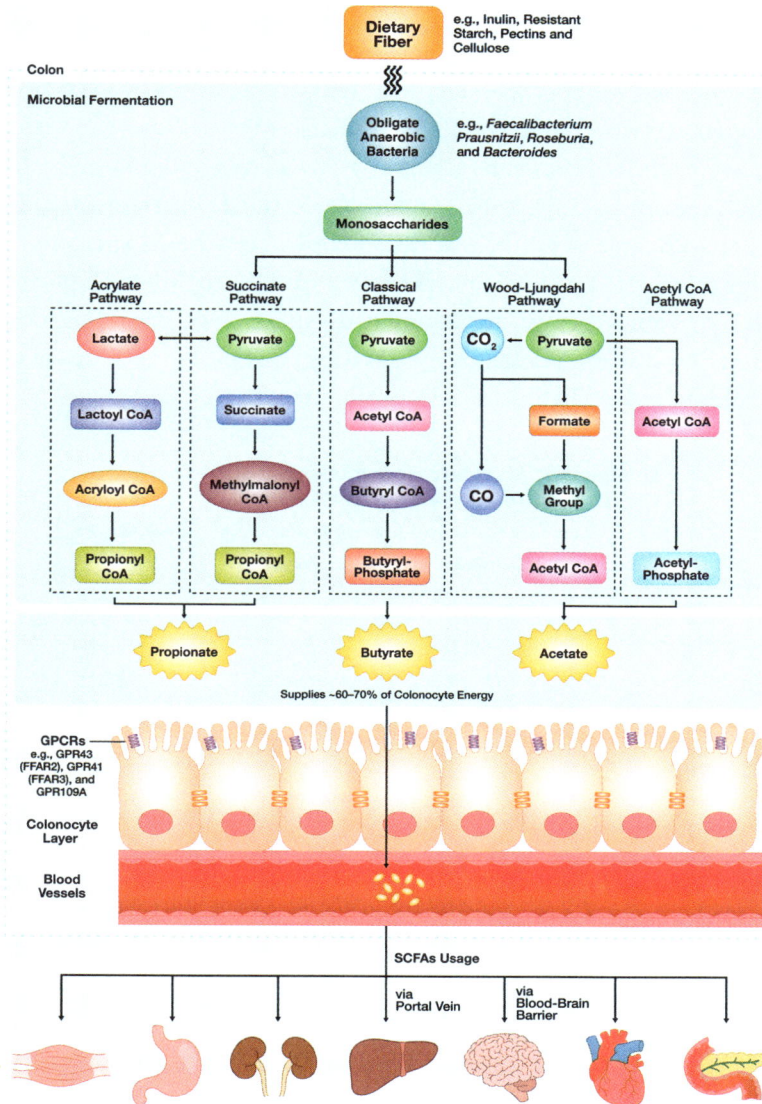

Fig. 34: Overview of microbial fermentation pathways and utilization of SCFAs by colonocytes, blood vessels, and systemic tissues, highlighting the role of obligate anaerobes in SCFA synthesis.

By the mid-twentieth century, scientists had identified specific anaerobic bacteria tied to SCFA production. Butyrate-producing Clostridia strains were noted for their anti-inflammatory effects. Early doctors observed that administering butyrate (for example, through enemas) could ease colitis symptoms, an early sign of its therapeutic potential. In the 1970s, the discovery of *Faecalibacterium prausnitzii* (initially misidentified as a *Fusobacterium*) was pivotal: It is abundant in healthy people and depleted in IBD patients, making it a key indicator of gut health. Meanwhile, *Bacteroides* species were recognized as versatile producers of acetate and propionate, equipped with many enzymes to break down diverse polysaccharides. These foundational studies collectively advanced our understanding of the microbial ecology behind SCFA production in humans.

Comparison of Dietary Fiber Intake and SCFA Levels
(Traditional vs. Modern Diets)

Diet Type	Estimated Fiber Intake	Dominant Microbial Genera	Health Outcomes
Paleolithic/Hunter-Gatherer	80–150 g/day (estimated)	High butyrate, propionate, acetate	Low incidence of metabolic & GI diseases
Traditional Agrarian	50–100 g/day	Robust SCFA production	Few IBS-, IBD- & obesity-related issues
Western Industrial	15–20 g/day	Reduced butyrate, higher acetate	Increased obesity, IBD, metabolic syndrome
Modern High-Fiber	25–40 g/day (guidelines)	Moderately high SCFA	Improved gut health, reduced inflammation

Summary of Microbial Composition & SCFA Levels

1. Paleolithic / Hunter-Gatherer Diet
- High fiber (80–150 g/day) High SCFA production
- Dominated by *Prevotella, Roseburia, Faecalibacterium*
- Butyrate-rich environment → Lower inflammation & metabolic disease risk

2. Traditional Agrarian Diet
- Moderate fiber (50–100 g/day) → Balanced SCFA levels
- Firmicutes & Bacteroidetes coexist in a stable microbiome
- Gut-health benefits → Lower risk of IBS, IBD, and obesity

3. Western Industrial Diet
- Low fiber (15–20 g/day) → SCFA imbalance
- Higher risk of inflammation, metabolic syndrome, and GI diseases
- *Bacteroides & Proteobacteria* dominate → Less butyrate, more acetate

4. Modern High-Fiber Diet
- Moderate fiber (25–40 g/day) → SCFA recovery
- Reintroduces butyrate-producing microbes
- Supports gut health & reduces inflammation risks

Table 2: Comparison of dietary fiber intake, dominant microbial genera, relative SCFA output, and health outcomes across historical and modern diets, underscoring the impact of fiber on gut health.

How the Western Diet Disrupts Gut Microbes and SCFA Production

It is not merely fiber deficiency that makes Western diets problematic. Western diets also contain elements that actively harm the gut microbiota and disrupt SCFA production, which is pivotal to our health. These features of an industrialized diet do two harmful things: They deprive beneficial fiber-fermenting bacteria of their fuel, and they create gut conditions hostile to microbial diversity and robust SCFA production. This disruption sets off a cascade of inflammatory and metabolic effects, compromising the symbiotic balance that traditional diets once supported.

Diets high in refined sugars (sucrose, high-fructose corn syrup, and other simple carbs) are mostly absorbed in the upper digestive tract, leaving very little for colonic microbes to ferment. Consuming a lot of sugar can cause certain sugar-loving microbes and yeasts (like *Candida*) to overgrow. This can make the colon environment too acidic for butyrate-producing anaerobic bacteria to survive, especially if there isn't enough fiber to buffer the acidity. The spikes of sugar, without fiber's stabilizing presence, cause boom-and-bust cycles in the microbiota, eroding its resilience. In contrast, ancestral high-fiber diets supported steady SCFA production and a stable microbial community.

All these dietary disruptors together render the Western gut an inhospitable place for fiber-dependent, SCFA-producing microbes. Studies show that those eating Western diets have far fewer key butyrate-producing bacteria (such as *Faecalibacterium prausnitzii*, *Roseburia intestinalis*, and *Eubacterium rectale*) compared to those eating fiber-rich agrarian or Mediterranean diets. Instead, Western microbiomes often have more *Bacteroides* species (adapted to protein- and fat-rich diets) and more Proteobacteria (a group that includes opportunistic pathogens). Fecal SCFA profiles in Western populations tend toward higher acetate and lower butyrate, and lower butyrate is a warning sign of a compromised colon lining. For example, a study comparing children in Italy (on a Western diet) with children in rural Burkina Faso (on a traditional high-fiber diet) found significantly lower total SCFA levels—especially butyrate—in the Western diet group, correlating with their lower fiber intake and fewer fiber-fermenting bacteria.

The hallmark of a fiber-deficient diet is a steep decline in SCFA production, which triggers a cascade of harmful effects that extend beyond the colon. A weakened gut barrier from low SCFAs becomes more permeable (leaky), allowing gut contents such as LPS to slip into the bloodstream. At the same time, fewer SCFAs mean less activation of certain receptors on immune cells (GPR41/43). In mice lacking one of these receptors (GPR43), inflammatory conditions such as colitis and arthritis are worse, suggesting that without SCFAs, the immune system is more prone to inflammation. Outside the gut, low fiber intake usually accompanies high-calorie diets, leading to obesity and inflammation in fat tissue. Butyrate and propionate normally help counter this by promoting regulatory T cells in fat that reduce inflammation. Without enough SCFAs, this protection is lost, and inflammation rises while insulin sensitivity drops.

Metabolic Endotoxemia: The Inflammatory Link to a Leaky Gut

Chronic low fiber intake leads to dysbiosis (an unhealthy gut microbial imbalance) that profoundly disrupts the gut-brain axis by reducing SCFA production, which is integral to neural and overall balance. One major consequence of diet-induced dysbiosis is that bacterial endotoxin (LPS) from the gut can leak into the bloodstream. This LPS crossing from the gut into circulation can have serious effects on the body.

Western-style high-fat, low-fiber diets have been shown to raise blood LPS levels two- to threefold in both rodents and humans, indicating a compromised gut barrier. LPS is a component of gram-negative bacterial cell walls. When the gut lining is weak, these bacteria or their products can penetrate the barrier, letting LPS slip into the blood. Once in the bloodstream, LPS triggers immune cells via the toll-like receptor 4 (TLR4), causing a release of pro-inflammatory cytokines (proteins that regulate immune responses) such as TNF-α, IL-1β, and IL-6—a state known as metabolic endotoxemia. In extreme cases, this can escalate to endotoxic septic shock, a severe condition of widespread inflammation causing low blood pressure and organ failure (responsible for millions of sepsis deaths globally each year).

Meanwhile, a leaky gut and circulating endotoxins keep the immune system in a chronically activated state, releasing a torrent of inflammatory mediators. This results in low-grade chronic inflammation throughout the body, a common thread in diseases such as atherosclerosis and type 2 diabetes. This systemic inflammation can also impact the brain: Cytokines from the blood can cross into the brain through weak points in the BBB or via active transport, and immune signals can travel through the vagus nerve to the brain. LPS itself can directly activate microglia (the brain's immune cells), leading to neuroinflammation.

In obesity, this metabolic endotoxemia manifests as activated microglia in the hypothalamus and elevated brain cytokines, which impair the brain's response to insulin and leptin, and contribute to further weight gain. It becomes a vicious cycle: Inflammation promotes obesity, and obesity fuels more inflammation. In summary, too few SCFAs and a disrupted gut microbiome have emerged as key links in the systemic and neural consequences of modern diets.

SCFA depletion also disrupts immune regulation. It leads to fewer regulatory T cells (Tregs) because SCFAs normally help promote their development (partly by HDAC inhibition). With fewer Tregs, the balance shifts toward inflammation, contributing to conditions such as asthma and autoimmunity. Epidemiological data tie low fiber intake to higher asthma rates, and animal models show propionate's protective role against allergic airway inflammation by boosting lung Tregs. Neurodegenerative disorders such as Parkinson's disease, Alzheimer's disease, and multiple sclerosis (MS) have all been associated with gut microbiome changes, including reduced SCFA levels. In a small MS study, adding propionate to standard therapy increased patients' Tregs and was associated with fewer relapses. In Alzheimer's patients, altered SCFA profiles are observed, which could worsen microglial activation and promote amyloid buildup over time.

To better understand how microbial imbalance and gut permeability might drive disease processes, researchers have turned to animal models. Groundbreaking work by researchers like Patrice Cani and others demonstrated that repeated infusion of low-dose LPS into mice causes key features of metabolic syndrome—weight gain, inflammatory immune cells invading fat tissue, and insulin resistance in the liver. This underscores LPS as a potent trigger of inflammation and metabolic problems. In the context of the gut-brain axis, LPS in the blood can reach the brain through areas with a weaker BBB or by transport mechanisms, activating microglia and causing neuroinflammation. Adequate SCFA production helps prevent this cascade by strengthening tight junctions and the mucosal defense system, thereby keeping LPS out.

Disturbances in the Gut-Brain Axis: How Dysbiosis and Low SCFAs Cause Problems

Chronic dietary fiber deficiency causes dysbiosis and significantly disrupts the gut-brain axis. This happens largely because low fiber means low SCFA production, and SCFAs are vital for keeping both gut and brain systems in balance. The imbalance affects the body and brain through multiple pathways, creating a cascade of effects on the host's physiology. A healthy, SCFA-rich microbiota helps regulate the HPA axis, modulating stress responses. Human studies support this assertion: Eating a high-fiber diet or taking probiotics can reduce perceived stress and improve mental well-being, likely by restoring SCFAs and gut-brain equilibrium.

SCFAs have neuroprotective effects. Notably, a small amount of butyrate can cross the BBB and strengthen it, as well as positively influence microglial cells in the brain. When dysbiosis leads to SCFA scarcity, the BBB can become weaker, allowing toxins and inflammatory mediators to enter the brain with increased ease, consequentially increasing the risk of neuroinflammation. Long-term lack of SCFAs, especially butyrate, is linked with colorectal disorders. For example, ulcerative colitis patients often have reduced fecal butyrate and fewer butyrate-producing microbes. Therapeutic butyrate enemas can reduce inflammation in distal colitis, and experiments transferring dysbiotic microbiota into germ-free mice have shown that this can cause colitis, implicating SCFA loss as a factor in colon inflammation.

Animal models show that butyrate keeps microglia in a calm, surveillant state (their normal, noninflammatory baseline), which counters the inflammatory response seen when SCFAs are lacking. In germ-free mice (which lack SCFAs), microglia remain immature and dysregulated, highlighting their dependence on microbial metabolites for proper development and function. Thus chronic SCFA depletion is a key link between dysbiosis and greater neurological vulnerability. The wide-ranging consequences of low SCFAs and dysbiosis include gut barrier dysfunction, immune dysregulation, metabolic imbalance, and disturbed gut-brain signaling, which are all implicated in a spectrum of chronic diseases. This complex interplay provides a strong rationale for therapies aimed at replenishing SCFA levels to correct dysbiosis and its harmful effects.

Butyrate's inhibition of HDAC enzymes also enhances brain-derived neurotrophic factor (BDNF) levels and synaptic plasticity in the brain (the brain's ability to rewire itself by forming new connections), adding to its therapeutic appeal. Certain diets boost butyrate-producing gut bacteria—for example, some ketogenic diets. This may help explain observed cognitive gains in Alzheimer's disease and fewer seizures in epilepsy patients on those diets. In animal models of multiple sclerosis (MS), butyrate promotes the repair of nerve insulation (myelin) by helping precursor cells mature, broadening the therapeutic scope of SCFAs.

Gut microbiota changes in people with autism spectrum disorder (ASD)—often including lower SCFAs—have been correlated with ASD symptoms, leading to various hypotheses about the gut-brain connection in autism. In one open-label study, children with ASD who received fecal microbiota transplantation (FMT) had increases in SCFAs and gut microbial diversity, and notably they showed improvements in gastrointestinal symptoms and core ASD symptoms. The benefits persisted two years after treatment. These results point to the gut-brain axis as an important therapeutic target in ASD.

Repair First, Then Rebuild: A New Path to Butyrate

When the colon has been chronically exposed to excess linoleic acid (LA), colonocytes are injured and the usual low-oxygen (anaerobic) environment is lost. That shift favors oxygen-tolerant, pro-inflammatory microbes over strict anaerobes—the very butyrate producers we're trying to nurture. In this damaged state, simply adding more fermentable fiber can be counterproductive: instead of yielding butyrate, dysbiotic bacteria may convert those substrates into endotoxin (LPS) and other inflammatory byproducts that worsen symptoms.

Direct butyrate supplementation is notoriously inefficient. Standard salts dissolve and absorb too early; tributyrin and even enteric coatings only partially solve the timing issue. The result is upper-gut exposure (odor, nausea, reflux) with very little reaching the colon— precisely where butyrate is needed to fuel colonocytes and restore barrier integrity.

The most effective entry point is not fiber or butyrate pills, but pasteurized (dead) *Akkermansia*. While marketed as "live," in reality, more than 99.9% of encapsulated cells perish before reaching the colon, either because the capsule breaks prematurely or because the oxygen-rich environment prevents survival. Far from a drawback, this turns out to be the advantage: dead *Akkermansia* still carries bioactive surface proteins such as Amuc_1100 and P9. These proteins deliver postbiotic effects—repairing the mucosal barrier, improving insulin sensitivity, and signaling metabolic resilience— even in the absence of viable colonization.

Taking dead *Akkermansia* only works optimally if the gut terrain is simultaneously improved. A low-LA diet reduces oxidative stress, lowers oxygen tension in the colon, and improves whole-body metabolism. Together, the postbiotic repair signals from *Akkermansia* and the systemic benefits of reduced LA create the conditions for the microbiome to begin recovering its anaerobic butyrate producers.

After one to two months of repair with pasteurized *Akkermansia* plus a low-LA diet, some individuals may experiment with encapsulated live strains. Even if they too largely perish, their transient presence and molecular debris can provide incremental benefits. The goal is not permanent colonization, but delivering additional postbiotic molecules in situ. This stage is about gentle layering, not sudden overhaul.

For both dead and live preparations, protection against upper-gut degradation is critical. The SOLARA system—glucomannan-based microencapsulation—resists digestion until the colon, where resident bacteria produce mannanases to break the shell and release the payload. This design maximizes the preservation of postbiotic proteins like Amuc_1100 and P9 and, if live bacteria are used, increases the odds of transient survival long enough to provide benefit.

Only once symptoms calm and colon physiology begins to normalize should fermentable fibers be reintroduced. The aim is not to bombard the gut with substrates, but to nurture newly viable anaerobes. Fibers should be added slowly, titrated to tolerance, and always paired with continued low-LA intake. At this stage, optional colon-targeted butyrate adjuncts may help, but the priority is restoring the body's own butyrate-generating ecosystem.

Protocol at a Glance: Restoring Butyrate

- **Step 1—Postbiotic Repair First:** Begin with pasteurized (dead) *Akkermansia*, ideally delivered via SOLARA encapsulation. Even though marketed as "live," nearly all cells are non-viable by the time they reach the colon. The benefit comes from their surface proteins (Amuc_1100, P9) and other postbiotic molecules, which signal gut repair and improve metabolic resilience.

- **Step 2—Pair with a Low-LA Diet:** Reducing dietary LA lowers oxidative stress, improves insulin sensitivity, and gradually restores the low-oxygen colonic environment needed for strict anaerobes to eventually thrive.

- **Step 3—Optional Live Trial:** After 1–2 months of repair and diet shifts, some individuals may introduce encapsulated live strains (including *Akkermansia* and select butyrate producers). Even if most die, their transient presence and molecular residues can add incremental benefit.

- **Step 4—Gradual Re-feed:** Only once gut tolerance improves should fermentable fibers be reintroduced slowly. The goal isn't fiber for its own sake, but nurturing the reborn anaerobic butyrate producers in an environment that can finally support them.

Key principle: Start with dead *Akkermansia* for repair, let the low-LA diet restore the terrain, then cautiously layer in live strains and fibers once the gut is ready.

Clinical Evidence of SCFA or Prebiotic Interventions

Study	Population	Intervention	Key Findings	Reference
Chambers et al. (2015)	Overweight adults	10 g/day Inulin-Propionate Ester (6 months)	Reduced weight gain, increased visceral fat, lowered satiety hormone release	[257]
Bourassa et al. (2021)	Autism spectrum disorder (ASD)	Prebiotic (8 g/day) for 12 weeks	Lowered body fat, increased SCFA production (especially butyrate)	[326]
Breuer et al. (2021)	Overweight subjects	Propionate-producing bacterial consortium	Lowered plasma cholesterol. Subjects had weight improvement.	[305]
Sonnenburg et al. (2022)	Ulcerative colitis patients	Butyrate enemas (100 mmol/L)	Some symptomatic relief. Small pilot study.	[283]
Vernia et al. (2021)	Crohn's disease patients	20 g/day Oligofructose-enriched inulin	Increase in fecal butyrate, and remission in a subset of patients	[249]

Table 3: Summary of clinical studies evaluating SCFA and prebiotic interventions, demonstrating therapeutic efficacy in metabolic and gastrointestinal disorders.

Fecal Microbiota Transplantation: Restoring Balance in the Gut Ecosystem

Fecal microbiota transplantation (FMT) is a treatment where an entire community of gut bacteria from a healthy donor is transferred to a patient with the aim of reestablishing SCFA-producing bacteria and a healthy microbiome. In patients with recurring *Clostridium difficile* (C. diff) infections, FMT has been extremely effective, likely because it reintroduces beneficial spore-forming Firmicutes that outcompete C. diff, along with other SCFA-producing bacteria that help suppress the pathogen. In ulcerative colitis patients, FMT has had moderate success—about 30 percent of patients achieve remission. Responders to FMT show greater microbial diversity and more SCFA-producing bacteria, and their post-FMT stool has higher butyrate levels, which are correlated with healing of the colon lining. Although FMT is still experimental for most conditions, it shows how recalibrating the microbiome toward an SCFA-rich state can be a powerful therapy.

Early case reports suggest FMT may even alleviate symptoms of Parkinson's disease, presumably by restoring SCFAs. Studies of the gut-brain axis highlight SCFAs' potential in neurodegenerative disorders, where dysbiosis and SCFA deficits are intertwined with disease progression. In experiments, transferring gut microbes from Parkinson's patients (who have fewer SCFA producers) into mice worsened the mice's motor symptoms, whereas giving those mice butyrate improved their movement and preserved their dopamine levels. This suggests that restoring SCFAs could benefit conditions such as Parkinson's.

These strategies can also be used for localized gut problems. For example, SCFA enemas can deliver relief directly to the lower colon in conditions such as ulcerative proctitis or radiation proctitis. Nightly enemas containing sodium butyrate (about 100 mmol/L in a 60–100 mL dose) have improved symptoms and even healed the colon lining in small groups of ulcerative colitis patients. However, larger trials have had mixed results, partly because it's hard for patients to maintain consistency with enemas long term. New innovations include special capsules that release SCFAs in the small intestine. These could potentially help with small intestinal bacterial overgrowth (SIBO) or boost GLP-1 release in the ileum, though these ideas are still in early development.

In summary, there are many approaches to increase SCFA levels: using prebiotics to nourish beneficial microbes, using probiotics or FMT to introduce good bacteria, and directly supplementing SCFAs (via capsules or enemas). Depending on the situation, these methods can range from preventive dietary fiber increases to disease-specific SCFA restoration therapies. All of these strategies aim to restore a healthier gut microbial balance, essentially regaining an ancient symbiosis within modern therapeutic practices.

Metabolic Syndrome and Type 2 Diabetes: Balancing Energy Through SCFAs

SCFAs have beneficial effects in people with metabolic syndrome and type 2 diabetes. They help regulate appetite, increase energy expenditure, and reduce inflammation. In obesity, the gut microbiome tends to shift toward simpler fermentation products and away from beneficial SCFAs such as butyrate.

Two SCFAs in particular—propionate and acetate—play distinct roles in regulating appetite and energy balance. Propionate can curb food intake by stimulating gut-brain circuits that increase GLP-1 (a hormone that signals fullness). Acetate also helps suppress appetite via the hypothalamus, though excessively high levels of acetate in the blood (beyond normal colonic production) might promote fat creation (lipogenesis). Delivering acetate to the colon (mimicking natural fermentation) avoids this fat-promoting effect.

In one study of overweight adults, increasing propionate production in the colon prevented weight gain, improved insulin sensitivity, and reduced visceral fat. In another small pilot study, obese insulin-resistant individuals took oral sodium butyrate (600 mg/day), and the results hinted at lower blood sugar and less inflammation. Ongoing trials (for example, one called PROP-ID) are testing propionate's role in preventing diabetes, highlighting SCFA-based interventions as a key tool in managing metabolic health.

Improving Mood and Brain Health with SCFAs

SCFAs have a significant impact on mood and cognitive function through multiple mechanisms, serving as a bridge between gut microbial activity and stable brain function. SCFAs can reduce systemic inflammation—a known factor in depression—thereby preventing an inflammatory environment that can disturb mood. Butyrate, in particular, promotes the growth of new neurons (neurogenesis) in the hippocampus (a part of the brain tied to memory and emotion) and boosts brain-derived neurotrophic factor (BDNF) levels. Patients with major depressive disorder have been found to have lower fecal SCFAs (especially butyrate) compared to individuals without depression, suggesting a link between the gut microbiome, inflammation, and depression. Experiments in mice have shown that butyrate produces antidepressant-like effects, supporting this theory.

Beyond specific conditions, SCFAs provide broad neuroprotection. They help safeguard neural integrity through both systemic effects and direct actions in the brain. By strengthening the gut barrier, SCFAs prevent inflammation-causing agents from leaking into the bloodstream and reaching the brain, thus preserving a healthy brain environment. SCFAs also stimulate the gut to produce hormones like GLP-1, which have neuroprotective properties. Some SCFAs even reach the brain themselves:

Acetate fuels astrocytes (brain cells that support and nourish neurons) and aids in producing neurotransmitter precursors. Butyrate supports the activity of glial cells, which help regulate brain inflammation and protect neurons. During low blood sugar or ketogenic conditions (like fasting or a keto diet), SCFAs become even more important as alternative energy sources for the brain, supporting neurons and helping glial cells maintain stability during stress or aging. Through all these avenues, SCFAs act as key guardians of brain health and resilience.

Therapeutic Considerations

Although lab studies and animal studies (as well as some observational human data) show great promise for SCFA therapeutic treatments, large, rigorous clinical trials are needed to confirm their efficacy and safety in people. There are some potential caveats to consider in acute situations. For example, during acute infections, too much fermentable fiber might feed harmful bacteria as well as helpful bacteria—though usually the beneficial SCFA-producers outcompete the harmful bacteria. In cancer, allowing bacteria to grow indiscriminately could be risky, so microbiome-based therapies must be applied with precision. Overall, boosting SCFAs offers an exciting opportunity to restore an evolutionary balance disrupted by modern diets. In doing so, we could potentially address a wide range of diseases affecting the gut, metabolism, and even the brain with a more holistic strategy.

SCFAs are central connectors between what we eat, our gut microbiota, and our physiology—with effects observed in tissues ranging from the intestinal lining to the brain's cerebral cortex. As evidence of their therapeutic promise grows, there are still many challenges to translating SCFA-focused interventions into everyday medical practice.

One major obstacle is ensuring effective delivery of therapeutic levels of SCFAs to the right part of the digestive tract. Scientists are exploring encapsulation technologies (such as capsules that survive stomach acid and release their contents in the colon) to improve delivery. We also don't yet know the optimal SCFA dosage for humans— high doses can cause gastrointestinal upset. To avoid this, researchers are testing strategies such as using tributyrin or attaching SCFAs to fiber (to target colon release). Enemas can bypass absorption and deliver SCFAs directly to the colon, but they only treat the lower bowel and are not practical for long-term use by most patients.

Summary of Current Challenges & Potential Solutions for SCFA Restoration

Challenge	Description	Potential Solutions	Next Steps
Delivery & Formulation	SCFAs absorbed prematurely, unpalatable (butyrate odor)	Enteric-coated capsules, SCFA prodrugs (IPE, tributyrin), better dosage studies	Optimize formulation, enhance palatability
Fiber Tolerance & Individual Variations	Some patients bloat with high-fiber intake; not all microbiomes respond similarly	Gradual fiber titration, personalized prebiotics, synbiotics, microbiome profiling	Develop personalized dietary strategies
Regulatory & Safety	Supplements vs. drugs: uncertain pathways for approval, off-target effects	Rigorous clinical trials, well-defined SCFA receptor agonists, regulatory clarity	Establish regulatory frameworks, safety studies
Comprehensive Approach Needed	SCFAs alone might not fix dysbiosis if lifestyle remains unchanged	Combine with diet overhaul, exercise, stress management, possibly other therapies	Integrate SCFA therapy into holistic health plans
Research Gaps	Optimal dose unknown, long-term effects unstudied, synergy with other interventions	Larger RCTs, multi-omics approach, standardized biomarkers (SCFA levels, etc.)	Conduct long-term studies, refine intervention models

Fig. 35: A summary of challenges and potential solutions for restoring SCFA levels, with proposed next steps for clinical translation.

Future Directions: Leading a Microbiome Revival with SCFA Therapies

The pivotal role of SCFAs in linking diet, gut microbes, and patient health heralds a transformative era of therapy. As research reveals more about SCFAs' health effects, future efforts must overcome current challenges to harness their full potential—moving beyond single-molecule supplements and toward restoring entire microbial ecosystems.

Emerging approaches prioritize rebuilding a functional microbiome with carefully designed microbial combinations (sometimes called "live biotherapeutics") rather than just giving SCFAs alone. These approaches use standardized mixes of beneficial gut bacteria (including key butyrate producers) to provide more consistent therapy than something like fecal microbiota transplantation (FMT), while ensuring a reliable dose of helpful microbes. These next-generation probiotics are meant to colonize and recalibrate the gut, representing an advanced step that could establish long-term microbial harmony.

While adding SCFAs directly can fix problems in the short term, it is equally as important to address the root causes of SCFA deficiency. Cutting down on unnecessary antibiotic use and other microbiome disruptors will help preserve SCFA-producing microbes. The concept of "rewilding" the gut—increasing exposure to diverse environmental microbes through outdoor activities or consuming traditional fermented foods—offers a holistic way to restore microbial diversity, especially early in life, when such interventions may have the greatest long-term impact. Optimizing SCFA therapies also requires good biomarkers (measurable signs in the body, such as specific molecules or patterns in stool or blood) to identify who will benefit and to measure success. In the future, precision nutrition might involve sequencing a patient's microbiome and tailoring prebiotic/probiotic regimens to boost SCFA output for that individual, an approach that is still in its infancy but likely to grow.

Chronic SCFA deficiency, particularly of butyrate, leads to mitochondrial dysfunction and thinning of the gut lining, impairing colon cell vitality. Future therapies could pair SCFA delivery with other nutrients—for example, vitamin D (to enhance the barrier) or glutamine (a vital fuel for gut cells)—to fully rehabilitate the gut lining. In severe dysbiosis, such as after intensive antibiotic treatments or in ICU patients on total parenteral nutrition (bypassing the gut), such combined interventions might prevent complications such as secondary infections resulting from impaired gut barrier function.

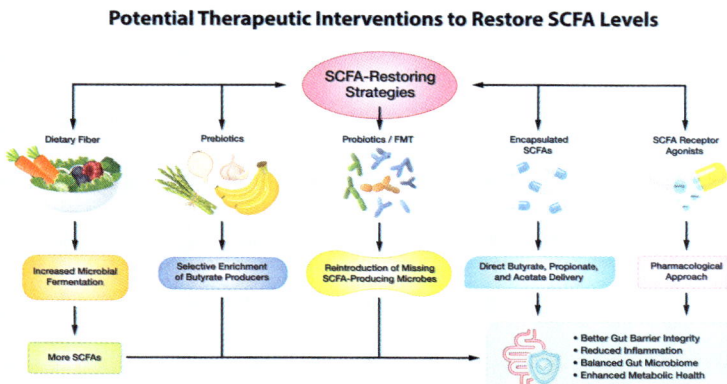

Fig. 36: Diagram of potential therapeutic interventions to restore SCFA levels, highlighting their impact on gut and systemic health.

Contemporary lifestyles have progressively eroded an ancient harmony between humans and the gut microbiome, an intricate balance built on dietary fiber, an array of gut microbes, and the SCFAs that sustain our physical and brain health. This review has traced a clear trajectory: from ancestral high-fiber diets that fostered microbial diversity and robust SCFA production, through the depletion of these metabolites amid industrialized dietary shifts, to the resulting cascade of health problems, and finally to innovative interventions aimed at reclaiming the lost benefits of SCFAs. All evidence points to a single truth: SCFAs are indispensable for maintaining a healthy colon, a balanced metabolism, and a harmonious interaction between the immune and nervous systems. Low levels of these metabolites are a common warning sign of dysbiosis and modern ailments, whether it's an inflamed gut in ulcerative colitis, insulin resistance in diabetes, or hyperactive microglia in neurodegeneration.

Reversing this harmful trend demands a multipronged therapeutic approach. Improving the diet is fundamental—gradually increasing intake of diverse fermentable fibers will nudge the microbiome toward higher SCFA production. Restoring the microbiota through probiotics, prebiotics, or fecal transplants can also help enhance the return of key SCFA-producing microbes. Yet the durability of such interventions depends on adherence; short-term fixes will fade if fiber-poor habits return. This underlines the need for public health initiatives and patient education to cement long-lasting dietary changes.

Viewing these metabolic issues through the gut-brain-axis lens enriches the discussion by showing the far-reaching effects of intestinal balance. Many modern diseases might find remedies in reestablishing a basic symbiosis. By once again nourishing our microbial partners, they will in turn nourish us with beneficial SCFAs. The onus is now on rigorous science, innovative thinking, and an informed public to help translate these insights into meaningful, real-world impact.

Gut Cure Figures

References: An Overview of the Gut Microbiome's Role in Health

This foundational paper draws on fifty-seven primary references, each carefully selected to reflect the most up-to-date understanding of how your gut microbiome interacts with metabolism, inflammation, and immune regulation. Most of these references were published in the last five years and include direct links to the full-text articles on PubMed. That means you don't have to take anyone's word for it; you can verify each claim and follow the trail of evidence as deeply as you want. Take control of your health and scan the QR code to review the original study yourself.

Index